# REFLEXOLOGY

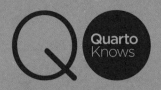

Inspiring | Educating | Creating | Entertaining

Brimming with creative inspiration, how-to projects, and useful
information to enrich your everyday life, Quarto Knows is a favorite
destination for those pursuing their interests and passions. Visit our
site and dig deeper with our books into your area of interest:
Quarto Creates, Quarto Cooks, Quarto Homes, Quarto Lives,
Quarto Drives, Quarto Explores, Quarto Gifts, or Quarto Kids.

First published in 2020 by Wellfleet Press,
an imprint of The Quarto Group
142 West 36th Street, 4th Floor
New York, NY 10018 USA
T (212) 779-4972 F (212) 779-6058
www.QuartoKnows.com

Wellfleet Press titles are also available at discount
for retail, wholesale, promotional, and bulk
purchase. For details, contact the Special Sales
Manager by email at specialsales@quarto.com or
by mail at The Quarto Group, Attn: Special Sales
Manager, 100 Cummings Center Suite 265D,
Beverly, MA 01915 USA.

10 9 8 7 6 5 4 3

ISBN: 978-1-57715-231-6

Group Publisher: Rage Kindelsperger
Creative Director: Laura Drew
Managing Editor: Cara Donaldson
Senior Editor: John Foster
Art Director: Cindy Samargia Laun
Cover and Interior Design: Ashley Prine,
    Tandem Books

Printed in China

This book provides general information on various widely known and widely
accepted images that tend to evoke feelings of strength and confidence. However, it
should not be relied upon as recommending or promoting any specific diagnosis or
method of treatment for a particular condition, and it is not intended as a substitute
for medical advice or for direct diagnosis and treatment of a medical condition by a
qualified physician. Readers who have questions about a particular condition, possible
treatments for that condition, or possible reactions from the condition or its treatment
should consult a physician or other qualified healthcare professional.

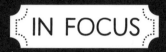

# IN FOCUS

# REFLEXOLOGY

## ❦Your Personal Guide❧

### TINA CHANTREY

WELLFLEET

PRESS

# CONTENTS

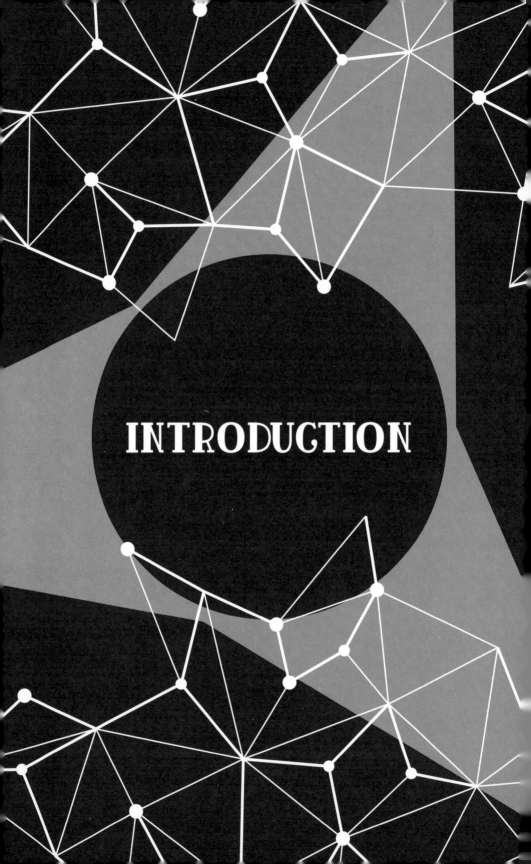

# INTRODUCTION

Reflexology is an ancient healing therapy that has been used for thousands of years. It can be learned and practiced by everyone. The benefits of this holistic art are myriad, ranging from the physical and emotional to the spiritual. In our technological age, dominated by screens and stress, the relaxing and healing benefits of reflexology have resulted in a surge in popularity for this therapy. At its root, reflexology refers to how one part of the body relates to another. Although many books focus only on using reflexology on the feet, this book covers hands, ears, and feet, giving readers and practitioners more choices when dealing with individual cases.

Well-being and happiness can often seem out of reach these days. But there is some good news: reflexology, which is a system of pressure and massage that is applied through the feet and hands, can provide relief from many of modern society's common ailments, including stress and anxiety. Good health is holistic, because our bodies and our minds need to cooperate to ensure well-being. The power of touch has always been used to heal, whether it's a parent massaging a newborn baby's feet or the mother of a child kissing it better after an accident.

This book is aimed at two types of readers. The first type is those of you who want to know about the subject for your own benefit and who may wish to give reflexology treatments to friends, relatives, and children. Unless the person has something wrong with their feet or some serious health condition, reflexology treatments should be completely harmless and probably very helpful.

The second type of reader is someone who might be considering taking up reflexology professionally. If that's you, you will need to study the subject further and to take a course of training, either in person or via the Internet. You will need to join the relevant reflexology organization in your country and to take out both public liability and professional indemnity insurance.

## The History of Reflexology

There were practices similar to reflexology in ancient Egypt as well as in China dating back as early as 2330 BCE. Modern reflexology was introduced to the United States in 1913 by William H. Fitzgerald, MD (1872–1942), who was an ear, nose, and throat specialist, and Edwin F. Bowers, a supporter of alternative medicine. Fitzgerald claimed that applying pressure to the feet created an anesthetic effect on other areas of the body. It was modified in the 1930s and 1940s by Eunice D. Ingham (1889–1974), a nurse and physiotherapist. Ingham claimed that the feet and hands were especially sensitive, and she mapped the entire body into "reflexes" on the feet. Modern reflexologists use Ingham's methods or similar systems that were later developed by the reflexologist Laura Norman.

# The Benefits of Reflexology

Reflexology is noninvasive, so it does not involve taking drugs or ingesting chemicals. It's a popular complementary therapy with many far-reaching benefits, and everyone can be helped by this ancient therapeutic art.

Sensors on the feet and hands are stimulated by applying the reflexology technique in order to improve the blood and energy circulation, give a sense of relaxation, and maintain homeostasis (balance).

Reflexology works on the energy field. It's believed that body parts can communicate using electromagnetic fields and that this communication can be blocked. Working on pressure points in the body may help restore the flow of energy, unblocking energy pathways. The manual application of pressure may also break up the lactic acid crystals that build up in the feet and hands, allowing energy to flow more efficiently. As each one of us is unique, results from reflexology can widely differ from one person to another.

## Reflexology Reduces Stress

Stress is a major factor in our lives and can be responsible for the development of many illnesses. It is impossible to avoid stress, but if it isn't managed, it can become a problem. Applying pressure to specific areas of the feet and hands induces a deep sense of relaxation, as the body's feel-good chemicals, known as endorphins, are produced. This helps the body cope with stress, and the more regular the treatments of reflexology are, the greater the benefit will be. Fears and anxieties will be soothed, and positive emotions will be promoted. Relaxation helps the body balance itself, promoting the flow of healing energy.

## Reflexology Improves Sleep

Whether you have a baby or toddler or whether you aren't getting regular sleep for some other reason, day-to-day life feels so much harder when you're sleep deprived. During sleep blood pressure drops, muscles relax, and blood supply increases. Tissue growth and repair occurs as growth hormones are released, which is essential for muscle development. Sleep helps us thrive by contributing to a healthy immune system, and it can also balance the appetite by helping regulate levels of the hormones ghrelin and leptin. Reflexology can help us relax, thereby promoting good-quality, deep sleep.

## Reflexology Improves Circulation

Applying pressure to your hands and feet will stimulate the circulatory system, which transports oxygen and vital nutrients around the body to the cells while also removing waste products. Stress can affect the circulation, so the relaxing effect of a reflexology treatment can be a huge boost. Good circulation also supports the immune system.

## Reflexology Stimulates Creativity

By promoting relaxation, reducing stress, and calming the mind, reflexology promotes clarity of mind. It's hard to allow ourselves to be creative when we are battling fatigue or stress. While stimulating mental energy and giving time to step away from busy, stress-filled lives, reflexology allows us to channel creative energy and refocus on issues, projects, or goals.

## Other Benefits

Reflexology can aid digestion, easing indigestion, irritable bowel syndrome, constipation, and flatulence along with food intolerances. It can help alleviate aches and pains, stiff joints, and menstrual problems. Not only this, reflexology can help improve focus and concentration. Overall, reflexology revitalizes the whole body, mind, and spirit.

# How Does Reflexology Work?

Reflexologists don't have a single answer to this question, but most believe that the areas on the foot correspond to areas on the body. Reflexology might be relatively new, but it has a close relative in palmistry, which is very ancient indeed, as there are Indian texts on the subject that go back over 5,000 years. Palmistry definitely shows links between various areas on the hands and different parts of the body, so it isn't surprising that some of the ideas and techniques have become adapted to create the basis of modern reflexology. Acupuncture and acupressure techniques are also involved in the thinking

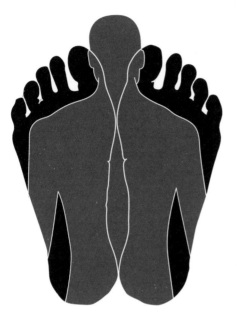

behind this treatment, with the idea that by manipulating areas on the feet, a practitioner can improve the health of people who suffer from various ailments.

There have been some concerns among medical professionals that people with potentially serious illnesses have tried to deal with them by means of reflexology, thus putting their lives at risk. This could be said of any therapy, which is why we call these therapies "complementary" as they seek to "complement" standard medical practice rather than replace it. People should be made aware of this at the time of the treatment, and they should be encouraged to keep up with their regular doctor visits.

Some reflexologists maintain that the blockage of an energy field, or an invisible life force, or qi, can prevent healing. Others suggest that the pressure the reflexologist gives to the feet may send signals to the nervous system or that the pressure may release chemicals such as endorphins that reduce stress and pain. Most believe that reflexologists can relieve stress and pain in other parts of the body through the manipulation of the feet. There is no scientific evidence for the existence of a mysterious life force, or qi, but that is the case for many spiritual and complementary concepts, yet they work.

## Reflexology and Practice

In the USA, reflexology is regulated on a voluntary basis by the Reflexology Association of America. In the UK, the Complementary and Natural Healthcare Council (CNHC) is its equivalent. Their members are required to meet standards of proficiency outlined by profession-specific boards. Charlatans are rare because it is a fact that most reflexologists are driven to give treatments in order to help and heal people, not to take their money in return for nothing

## Tip

••••◆◆◆◆◆••••

Avoid carrying out reflexology on those who have numb areas on the feet due to diabetes, deep vein thrombosis, phlebitis, osteoarthritis, or cellulite on the feet or legs, or those who have had strokes or are pregnant. Avoid treating those who have fractures, unhealed wounds, foot or leg ulcers, or gout.

worth having. Nevertheless, if you decide to use the services of a reflexologist or, indeed, any kind of therapist and your intuition tells you this person is not the right fit for you, you must always listen to your inner voice.

## Some Important Things to Bear in Mind

- People should wait an hour after the treatment before eating.
- Pregnant women should *not* request a treatment; they should just have a massage instead.
- People should drink water after the treatment as this will help clear toxins out of the body and clear any lactic acid that may build up or get released during the treatment.
- People should consult a doctor if they have any foot problems, such as an injury, numb areas of the foot, blood vessel disease, clots, or varicose veins.

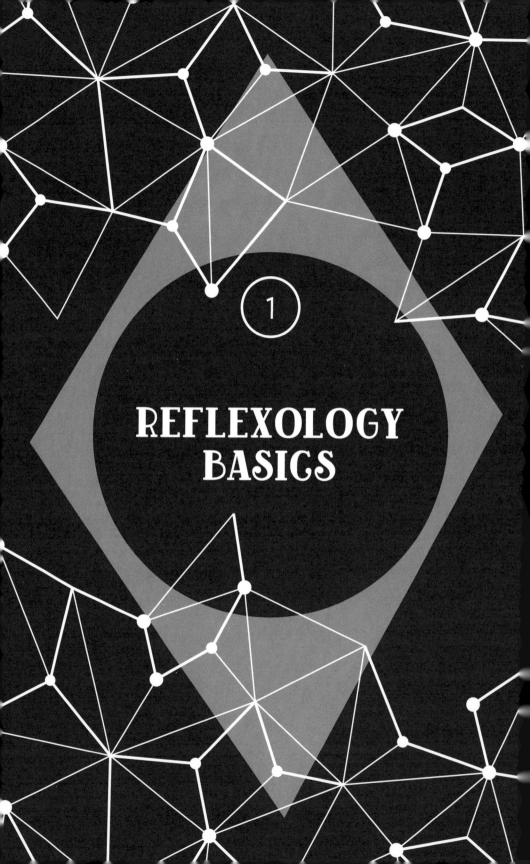

1

# REFLEXOLOGY BASICS

As mentioned in the introduction, reflexology is a noninvasive therapy based on touch. Each foot and ankle has twenty-six bones; thirty-three joints; more than one hundred muscles, tendons, and ligaments; and thousands of nerves. Through touch and gentle pressure during reflexology, these nerves are stimulated, helping to relax the body and allowing its own self-healing mechanism to function as best it can. Reflexology aims to remove the energy blockages that occur in the body due to a poor diet, insufficient exercise, or stress, whether they are due to work, relationships, or other life events. Reflexology opens the channels for natural healing and restores balance. It is beneficial to all ages, from babies onward.

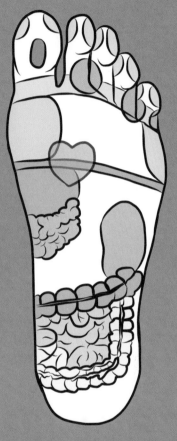

An artistic representation of the areas of the feet as treated by reflexology.

## Feet and Reflexology

Many of us never touch our own feet, even though they do so much for us every day, but with the advent of touch from a practitioner, the healing powers of the body can be activated. Since the times of the ancient Egyptians, about 4,000 years ago, there are records of people working on feet to promote good health.

Reflexology is based on energy zones that run through the body, as well as reflex areas in the feet that correspond to all the major organs, tissues, and glands. When Dr. William Fitzgerald developed the modern form of reflexology, he divided the body into ten equal longitudinal energy areas: five relating to the right half of the body and five to the left half.

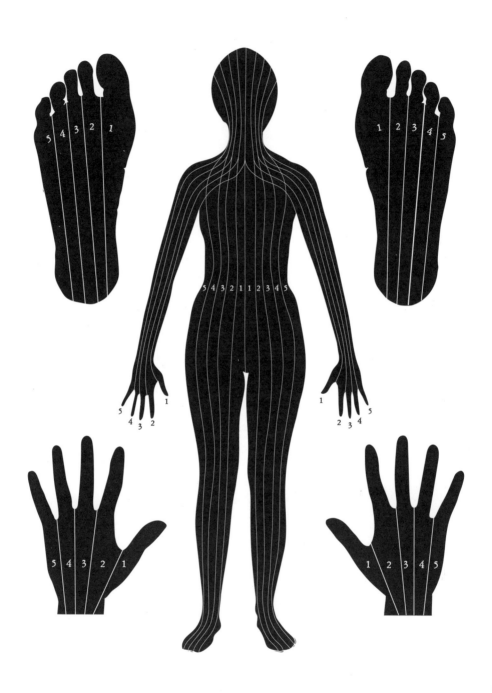

The longitudinal zones.

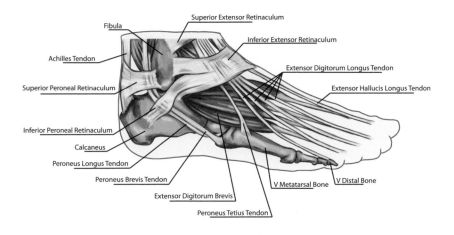

The anatomy of the foot.

Fitzgerald's work inspired physiotherapist Eunice Ingham, who mapped the entire body on the feet during the 1930s, indicating the most sensitive and responsive areas of the body. As we will see in chapter 2, each foot and hand contains a mini map of the body. Through pressure on reflex points on each map, the whole body can be stimulated, encouraging balance between the different body systems.

Research on this therapy is constantly being updated, but studies have shown that reflexology can assist with reducing pain and anxiety. It does not treat specific diseases, but it can bring about a change in the body that enables it to heal.

# The Healing Crisis

No two people will react in the same way to reflexology—you or a recipient may experience different sensations and responses each time you have a session. When practicing reflexology, you should be aware of some common reactions, one of which is called the "healing crisis."

After a reflexology session, some people experience symptoms such as pain, joint aches, muscle cramps, mood swings, fatigue, or a sudden heavy coldness. For many, these symptoms can get worse before they start to diminish, which may not start to happen until after several sessions. Anyone receiving work on their body, from deep tissue work to energy work or reflexology, can experience a healing crisis, and for some it can feel frightening.

A healing crisis occurs because the body is trying to eliminate toxins at a faster rate than they can be disposed of. It's a positive sign that the treatment is working, and the body is trying to cleanse itself of toxins and imbalances. There is no specific time frame for a healing crisis to occur; some will experience it during the session, but others find it comes on afterward and may give them symptoms for several days.

The impurities are squeezed out of the tissues of the body and they flow into the bloodstream, causing a toxic reaction until the body has eliminated them. Even though it may not feel pleasant, a healing crisis is a good sign, because it signals that a cleansing process is under way.

The same thing happens with other therapies, including weight-loss groups. It is not unusual for group members to be fine for the first three weeks, and then at week four, their weight loss stalls, and they feel off and somewhat depressed. If the group leader explains that this is normal and that they should work through it, they stay in the group and continue to lose weight in a slow and steady manner.

Some people experience an emotional release during or after reflexology, because emotions and memories stored in the muscles rise to the surface. When negative feelings are suppressed, the body becomes a storehouse for them, so releasing feelings of grief and anger is common during a treatment, and some people may suddenly cry, laugh, cough, twitch, or get a cramp or headache.

# Support During a Reflexology Session

At the start of any session, be aware that you or someone else may experience a healing crisis. Anyone experiencing a healing crisis should drink plenty of water to aid the body in eliminating toxins. When fatigue is severe, the first priority should be sleep, as this is the best way for the body to recover. If an emotional release occurs, the best thing to do is be open to this, be aware of feelings, and try to remain grounded. Rest assured that the feelings being experienced are all right and that this is the body's way of letting go of emotion. Most symptoms disappear within twenty-four hours, but if you or your recipient experiences a prolonged healing crisis, it would be best to then seek the help of a professional counselor. And remember, not everyone experiences a healing crisis—it doesn't need to occur for reflexology to be recognized as a success!

# When *Not* to Practice Reflexology

Before you touch your feet or someone else's, a simple, visual scan will give you vital clues to the current state of health. Certain conditions need extra care and consideration. Reflexology should not be practiced if any of the following conditions are present. When in doubt, seek a doctor's advice and/or permission to give treatment.

- A contagious condition such as ringworm, impetigo, or chicken pox
- An open sore or wound
- Pregnancy with a history of miscarriage
- Diabetes
- A pacemaker
- Over areas of broken veins
- Over varicose veins
- Over recent surgery
- Ongoing medical treatment for a serious condition
- Obvious signs of being under the influence of drugs or alcohol

**Diabetics** need to take extra care with scratches and wounds, because diabetes can make them extra susceptible to infection. Some diabetics suffer with nerve damage in the feet (neuropathy), which causes numbness, so they don't notice when other damage occurs. If you are unsure, treat a diabetic's hands, which tend to have more feeling than the feet due to less nerve damage and better circulation.

**Gout** affects the toes and can be extremely painful, causing swelling, inflammation, and throbbing. This condition tends to affect men more than women and results from a buildup of uric acid in the blood. Reflexology can help this condition by encouraging detoxification.

**Chilblains** occur in cold weather when small blood vessels become inflamed and can result in red swellings on both fingers and toes. Sufferers often feel a burning or itching sensation in the affected areas. In severe cases, chilblains can develop into blisters or open sores. Reflexology should *never* be performed on any blistered, broken, or sore skin. However, when chilblains are less severe, reflexology may give relief, as it improves the body's general circulation.

**Athlete's foot** is a fungal infection between the toes. It is advisable to do reflexology on the hands if you or a recipient have this condition.

**Edema** can lead to a buildup of fluid in the tissues of the ankles and feet, causing swelling and pain. Treat the hands for reflexology until the condition has improved, when you can start treating the feet as long as you do so gently. Encourage sufferers to remain hydrated, and ask them to check that their urine is the color of straw rather than brown. Also ensure they talk to their doctor about their condition.

As you become more experienced, you will be able to observe feet and recognize warning signs that the body is unbalanced. When you check the feet, are they pale and cold to the touch? If so, this could suggest poor circulation or sometimes the effects of the medicines that the person is taking. Dry skin may indicate dehydration or a digestive problem.

# Reflexology and Weight Loss

There are some claims that reflexology can help those who want to lose weight, because it can trigger the body's ability to eat the right foods and to use up some of the excess fat stored in it. The main way reflexology may be able to help people lose weight is through promoting their sense of overall well-being. Combined with regular exercise, as well as eating a healthy, balanced diet, reflexology may help them stay on track. By sleeping better and feeling less stressed, they are more likely to exercise, stick to a healthy diet, and achieve their weight-loss goals.

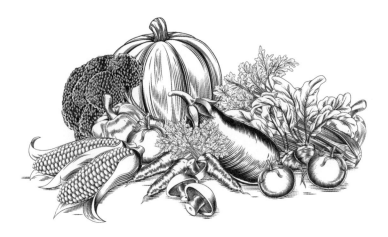

## Other Benefits

Many people turn to reflexology to help them stop smoking, reduce their alcohol intake, and cope with phobias. Feeling happier within affects health, relationships with others, and a person's ability to adapt to stress.

## A Quick Summary

Reflexology works on the glands and soft tissues; it stimulates nerve functions, increases energy levels, and improves circulation and the action of the central nervous system. It can prevent migraines, help the body's natural healing mechanism to clear infections, alleviate sleep disorders, and help with depression.

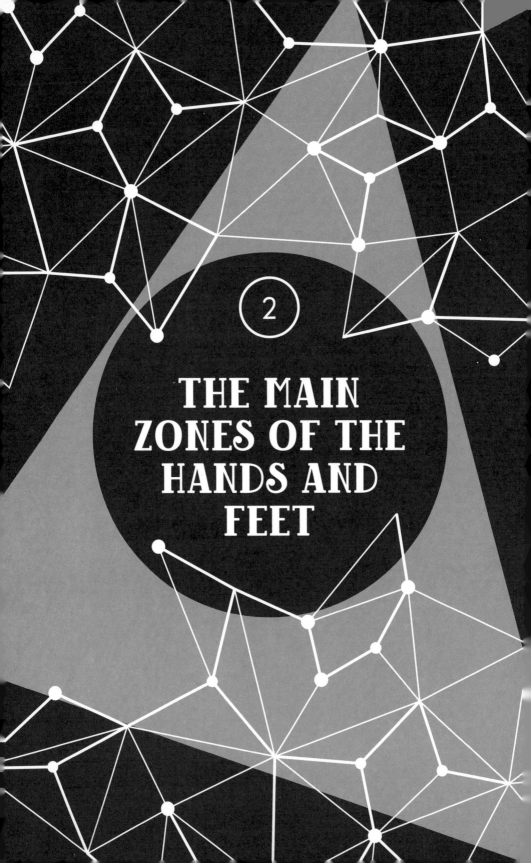

# 2

# THE MAIN ZONES OF THE HANDS AND FEET

There are many therapies that work with the energy zones, or meridians. Originally, Dr. William Fitzgerald divided the body into ten energy zones, five on each side of the spine, running from the big toe up through the head. The hands are also zoned, with Zone 1 starting at the thumb. These zones run longitudinally as well as pass through the body from back to front, and they are similar to the meridians in acupuncture. Along these meridians are acupuncture points that relate to different systems. The zones on the soles of the feet mirror the body, and each one is a channel for life energy that is known as *chi* or *qi*. Blockages along them will cause problems in the associated body area.

A reflex zone illustrates the interconnection of the different parts of the body. Pressure applied to a region may help a specific organ or particular area in order to alleviate the pain and symptoms of a disease. Each zone interconnects with several different parts of the body, so working on any zone through the application of pressure by your thumbs and fingers will affect the entire zone.

## Tip

Although the spellings of *qi* and *chi* might be different, the pronunciation of both is "chee."

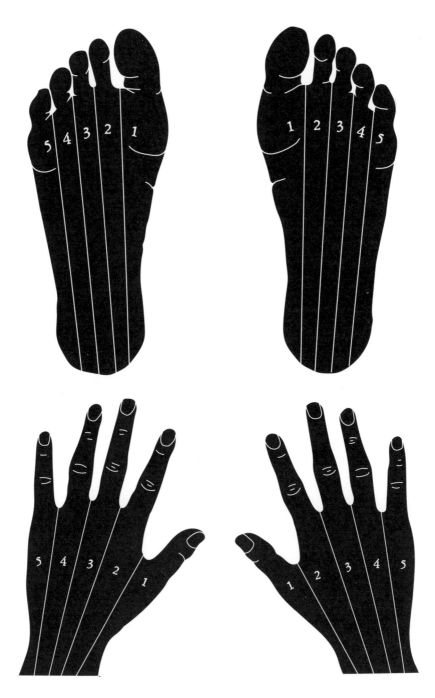

The zones of the feet and hands.

# The Left Foot and Its Corresponding Organs

## ZONE LINE 1
### LEFT THUMB AND BIG TOE ON LEFT FOOT

Pituitary, pineal, brain, hypothalamus, thyroid, sinuses, nose, larynx, trachea, esophagus, tongue, thymus, heart, spine, pancreas, breast, small intestine, large intestine, and prostate.

## ZONE LINE 2
### LEFT INDEX FINGER AND SECOND TOE

Brain, eye, adenoids, lung, heart, stomach, spleen, pancreas, breast, small intestine, and large intestine.

## ZONE LINE 3
### LEFT MIDDLE FINGER AND THIRD TOE

Brain, eye, lung, breast, stomach, spleen, pancreas, kidney, adrenal gland, small intestine, and large intestine.

## ZONE LINE 4
### LEFT RING FINGER AND FOURTH TOE

Brain, eye, lungs, breast, large intestine, and ovaries.

## ZONE LINE 5
### LEFT LITTLE FINGER AND FIFTH TOE

Left ear.

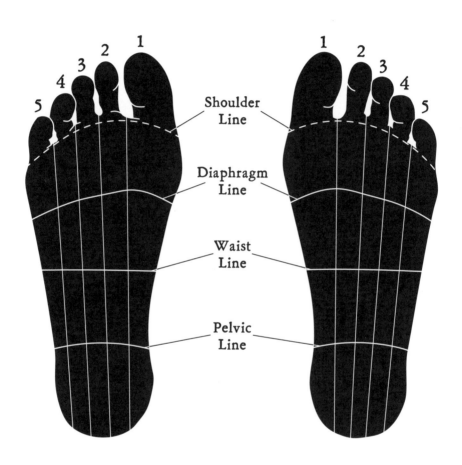

The zones and lines of the feet.

# The Right Foot and Its Corresponding Organs

## ZONE LINE 1
### RIGHT THUMB AND BIG TOE ON RIGHT FOOT

Pituitary, pineal, brain, hypothalamus thyroid, sinuses, larynx, nose, trachea, tongue, esophagus, thymus, heart, spine, pancreas, small intestine, large intestine, and prostate.

## ZONE LINE 2
### RIGHT INDEX FINGER AND SECOND TOE

Brain, eye, lung, breast liver, small intestine, large intestine, and adenoids.

## ZONE LINE 3
### RIGHT MIDDLE FINGER AND THIRD TOE

Brain, eye, breast, liver, gallbladder, kidney, small intestine, large intestine, and adrenal gland.

## ZONE LINE 4
### RIGHT RING FINGER AND FOURTH TOE

Brain, eyes, main lymphatic duct, breast, liver, lung, large intestine, ileocecal valve, and appendix.

## ZONE LINE 5
### RIGHT LITTLE FINGER AND FIFTH TOE

Right ear.

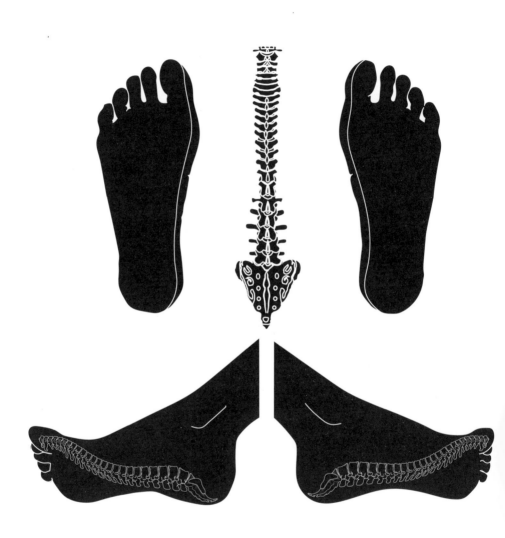

The spine reflex.

## The Inner Foot

When you look at your feet, you will see a natural curve on the inside of each foot which creates a reflex that corresponds to the spine. The area from the base of the big toenail to the base of the toe corresponds to the cervical vertebrae that are found in the neck. The large bulge beneath the big toe corresponds to the thoracic part of the spine, which runs from the shoulders to the waist line. The area between the middle of the foot and the heel (waist line to pelvic line) relates to the lumbar vertebrae. The area from the heel line to the base of the heel refers to the sacrum and coccyx. The reflex area for the bladder is just below the lumbar region on the inside of each foot.

## The Outer Foot

The outer edge of the feet corresponds to the outer parts of the body, which are the shoulders and upper arms (base of toes to diaphragm line); elbows, forearms, wrist, and hand (diaphragm line to waist line); and legs, knees, and hips (from the fifth metatarsal to the heel line).

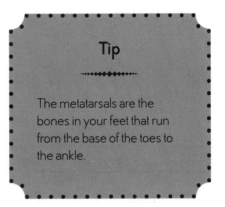

### Tip

The metatarsals are the bones in your feet that run from the base of the toes to the ankle.

## The Ankle Area

The area around the ankle on each foot relates to the pelvic area and reproductive organs. The outer ankle area contains reflex points for the ovary/testicle. The inner ankle contains points for the uterus/prostate, vagina/penis, and bladder. A narrow band running from below the anklebone across the top of the foot from one anklebone to the other holds the reflex points for the fallopian tubes, lymph drainage area in the groin, vas deferens, and seminal vesicle.

The general pelvic/rectum/prostate/uterus/sciatic nerve area begins six inches above the anklebone and runs down to the uterus/prostate point found below the ankle. The sciatic nerve travels down both sides of the leg, then across the heel, but as this is the nerve and not a reflex area, it can be sensitive.

✳ ✳ ✳

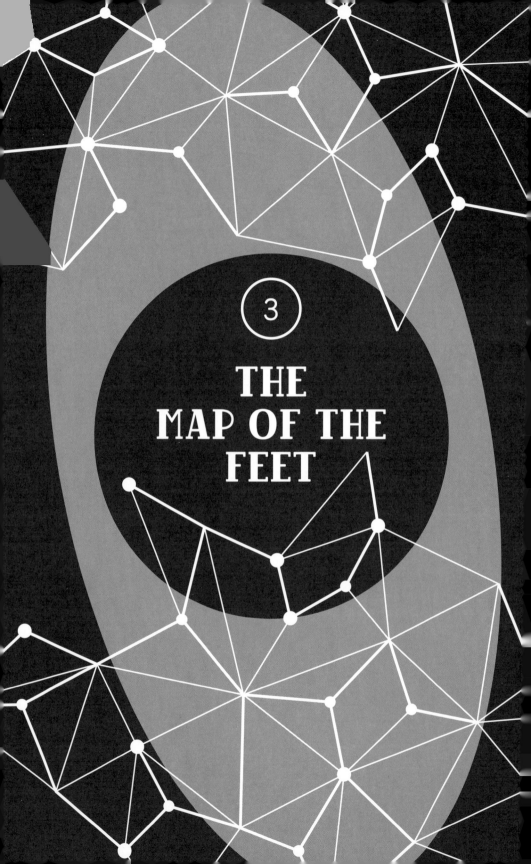

3

# THE MAP OF THE FEET

Now that you're familiar with the zones of the feet, let's take a more detailed look at how those zones relate to other parts of the body. Blocked energy can affect the organs and systems that lie within that zone, so by restoring balance in the body systems, reflexology is helping the body achieve a state called *homeostasis.* Any area of the body can be located on the map of the feet.

A foot reflexology chart shows the location of all the reflex points on the feet. Applying pressure on these points can help heal ailments related to that part of the body. It's worth taking some time to study a map of the feet to help you learn where the reflex points on them correspond to different parts of the body. All of the major organs of the body are located on a chart. Organs located on the left side of the body are found on the left foot, whereas those located on the right side of the body are associated with the right foot. For example, the liver is located on the right side of the body, so applying reflexology to the right foot may help alleviate liver problems.

## The Body as Shown on the Map of the Feet

If you're starting out with foot reflexology, familiarize yourself with a sole chart (see page 30). This doesn't give information about the tops or sides of feet, but it is fairly easy to learn and a good starting point to understand how the foot relates to different parts of the body.

You will see that the toes are connected to the head, brain, ears, eyes, pineal gland, pituitary gland, and neck. More details of how each part of the foot corresponds to a body part, and how working on this reflex can help treat any health conditions related to that body part, can be found after the charts of the sole, top, inside, and outside of the feet.

## THE MAP OF THE FEET

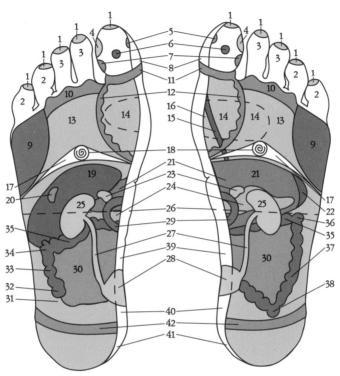

1. Brain
2. Sinuses, outer ear
3. Sinuses, inner ear, inner eye
4. Temple
5. Pineal gland, hypothalamus
6. Pituitary gland
7. Side of the neck
8. Cervical spine C1 to C7
9. Shoulder, arm
10. Neck to eye area, inner ear, eustachian tube
11. Neck, thyroid, parathyroid, tonsils
12. Bronchial, thyroid area
13. Chest, lungs
14. Heart
15. Esophagus
16. Thoracic spine T1 to T12
17. Diaphragm
18. Solar plexus
19. Liver
20. Gallbladder
21. Stomach
22. Spleen
23. Adrenals
24. Pancreas
25. Kidneys
26. Waist line
27. Urethra tube
28. Bladder
29. Duodenum
30. Small intestine
31. Appendix
32. Ileocecal valve
33. Ascending colon
34. Hepatic flexure
35. Transverse colon
36. Splenic flexure
37. Descending colon
38. Sigmoid colon
39. Lumbar spine L1 to L5
40. Sacral spine
41. Coccyx
42. Sciatic nerve

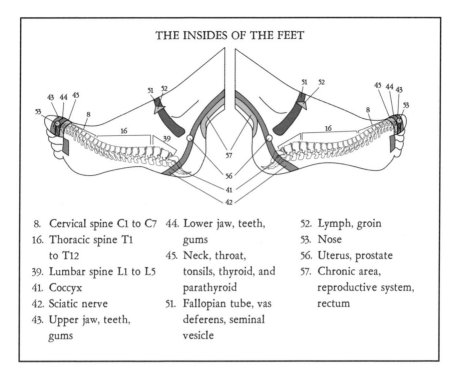

THE INSIDES OF THE FEET

8. Cervical spine C1 to C7
16. Thoracic spine T1 to T12
39. Lumbar spine L1 to L5
41. Coccyx
42. Sciatic nerve
43. Upper jaw, teeth, gums
44. Lower jaw, teeth, gums
45. Neck, throat, tonsils, thyroid, and parathyroid
51. Fallopian tube, vas deferens, seminal vesicle
52. Lymph, groin
53. Nose
56. Uterus, prostate
57. Chronic area, reproductive system, rectum

# Correspondences to the Insides of the Feet

The above chart of the insides of the feet, the part of the foot that faces inward toward the other foot, shows in more detail how this area relates to corresponding body parts. From the bottom of the of the foot, near the ankle, to the top of the big toe represents the spine. Once you spend some time working on your own feet, you will notice how the insides of each foot have the same basic shape of the spine, with similar curves. Under the waist line there is a puffy mound on the inside of the foot, which is connected to the bladder.

The inside of the toes is connected to the jaw, teeth, gums, and neck. A strip below the ankle relates to the reproductive system.

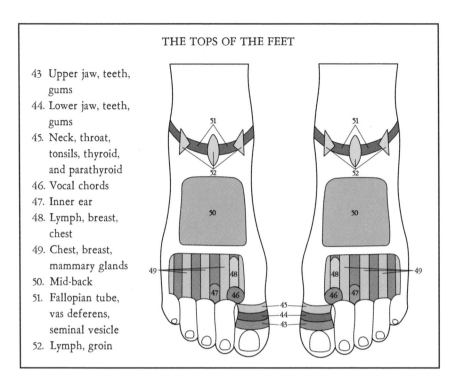

THE TOPS OF THE FEET

43 Upper jaw, teeth, gums
44. Lower jaw, teeth, gums
45. Neck, throat, tonsils, thyroid, and parathyroid
46. Vocal chords
47. Inner ear
48. Lymph, breast, chest
49. Chest, breast, mammary glands
50. Mid-back
51. Fallopian tube, vas deferens, seminal vesicle
52. Lymph, groin

# Correspondences to the Tops of the Feet

The very tops of the feet correspond to the chest and the lymphatic system, which is part of the immune system. Lymph filters toxins and other waste products from the body.

# Correspondences to the Outsides of the Feet

The accompanying chart of the outsides of the feet—the part that faces away from the body—shows what area of the body corresponds to these reflex areas. The side of the foot above the heel relates to the knees and hips. The side of the foot below the waist line relates to the elbow, and the area underneath the smallest toe relates to the shoulder.

The soles of the feet are divided into three areas. The top third incorporates the toes, which relate to the head and neck, and the balls of the feet, which relate to the heart, chest, thymus, lungs, and shoulders. The next section down,

## OUTSIDE VEW OF THE LEFT FOOT AND INSIDE VIEW OF THE RIGHT FOOT

### Outside Left View

9. Shoulder, arm
42. Sciatic nerve
43. Upper jaw, teeth, gums
44. Neck, throat, tonsils, thyroid, parathyroid
45. Neck, throat, tonsils, thyroid, and parathyroid
46. Vocal chords
47. Inner ear
48. Lymph, breast, chest
49. Chest, breast, mammary glands
50. Mid-back
51. Fallopian tube, vas deferens, seminal vesicle
52. Lymph, groin
57. Chronic area, reproductive, rectum
58. Leg, knee, hip, lower back
59. Hip, sciatic area
60. Ovary, testes

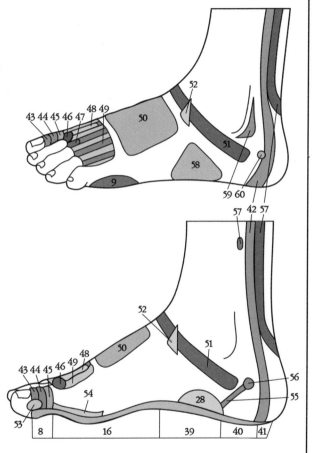

### Inside Right View

8. Cervical spine C1 to C7
16. Thoracic spine T1 to T12
28. Bladder
39. Lumbar spine L1 to L5
40. Sacral spine

41. Coccyx
53. Nose
54. Thymus
55. Penis, vagina
56. Uterus, Prostate

## OUTSIDE VIEW OF THE RIGHT FOOT AND INSIDE VIEW OF THE LEFT FOOT

**Outside Right View**

50. Mid-back
51. Fallopian tube, vas deferens, seminal vesicle
52. Lymph, groin
57. Chronic area, reproductive system, rectum
58. Leg, knee, hip, lower back
59. Hip, sciatic area
60. Ovary, testes

**Inside Left View**

8. Cervical spine C1 to C7
16. Thoracic spine T1 to T12
28. Bladder
39. Lumbar spine L1 to Lt
40. Sacral spine
41. Coccyx
53. Nose
54. Thymus
55. Penis, vagina
56. Uterus, Prostate

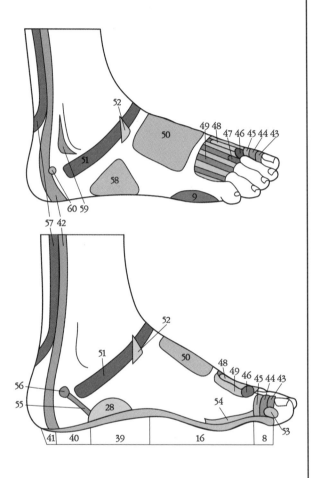

separated from the top third by what reflexologists call the "diaphragm line," down to the "waist line," relates to the liver, gallbladder, stomach, kidneys, adrenal glands, pancreas, and spleen.

You can find the "waist line" by locating the bone that protrudes from the outside of the foot, which is known as the "metatarsal notch." The area from the diaphragm to the waist line relates to the liver, gallbladder, stomach, kidneys, adrenals, pancreas, and spleen.

The pelvic line encompasses the area beneath the heel of the foot; this line is between the inside and outside of the anklebone. The inside and outside of the anklebone are reflex areas for the bladder, small intestine, and large intestine. The heel relates to the sciatic nerve and pelvic area.

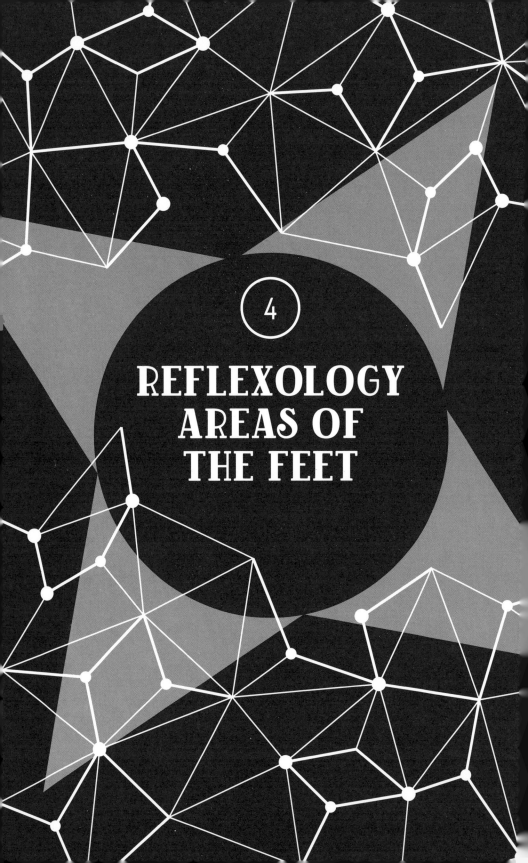

4

# REFLEXOLOGY AREAS OF THE FEET

At this stage, it's important to begin to grasp the way the body and its interrelating systems and organs work.

## The Reflexes Found on the Toes

The toes relate to the head, brain, eyes, ears, nose, sinuses, face, mouth, neck, and upper shoulders. The big toe relates to the head, containing the reflex point for the pituitary gland, pineal gland, hypothalamus, brain, temples, upper and lower jaw, gums, teeth, throat, thyroid and parathyroid, and the seven cervical vertebrae.

### The Brain

The brain consists of the brain stem, which controls vital functions such as breathing, blood pressure, and pulse. The cerebellum controls sleep, breathing, circulation, and consciousness, and it coordinates movement and balance. It is divided into the right and left hemisphere, which control movement and communication. The right side controls the left side of the body in addition to creativity, intuition, artistic ability, and nonverbal communication. The left side of the cerebellum controls the right side of the body in addition to speech, logic, writing, language, mathematical skills, and analytical thinking. Both hemispheres have jobs to do, so they both need to be used. When a stroke disables one hemisphere, it affects the way the body works.

### The Pituitary Gland

This gland, about the size of a pea, sits behind the eyes and nose. It controls the release of hormones in the body, affecting the endocrine system. Known as the "master gland," it controls several other hormone glands in the body including the thyroid, adrenals, ovaries, and testicles. Growth, sexual development, pregnancy, metabolism, energy levels, and temperature are just some of the body's functions that are influenced by the pituitary gland.

## The Sinuses

These air-filled cavities in the head, situated behind the cheekbones and forehead, filter the air that is breathed in as well as act as a draining system for the head. They also help protect the face in case of trauma, insulate against rapid temperature changes in the nose, and provide immunological defense. Infected sinuses cause head pain, and problems in these areas make breathing through the nose difficult.

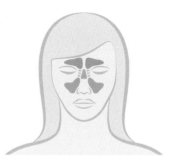

## The Hypothalamus

This gland regulates the autonomic nervous system, controlling emotions, reactions, body temperature, and appetite. It has the same reflex point as the pineal gland. It acts as a communications center for the pituitary gland, sending messages to this gland in the form of hormones, via the bloodstream and down the pituitary stalk.

## The Pineal Gland

This small gland in the brain responds to levels of daylight to produce melatonin, which affects circadian rhythms, such as when we go to sleep and wake up. It's sometimes known as the "third eye," and its reflex point is located in Zone 1, on the inner side/top of each big toe.

## The Thyroid

The thyroid gland is part of the endocrine system and controls the metabolism, which affects energy levels. It's located on the front of the neck, and its reflex area is found at the base of each big toe. Hypothyroidism means a low-functioning thyroid, which can cause the metabolism to slow down. It leads to weight gain and water retention, and sufferers often have distinctively prominent eyes. Hyperthyroidism means an overactive thyroid, which can cause the functions in the body to run too fast. Someone suffering from this condition loses weight easily.

## The Parathyroid

Found around the thyroid, these four tiny glands located in the neck affect both calcium and phosphate levels that are essential for muscle function. They do this by secreting a protein called parathyroid hormone (PTH).

## The Cervical Vertebrae

The neck is made up of seven cervical vertebrae, with the seventh one (which can be felt at the base of the neck) being the last and most prominent. Its reflex point is found at the base of the big toe of both feet in Zone 1. The small toes each contain one zone and are used for head and neck issues such as sinusitis, hearing problems, and neck tension. People who have suffered head or brain injuries or strokes can benefit from having the tips of all the toes massaged. The ridge at the base of the toes is worked on as a "helper area" for eyes, ears, and eustachian tube disorders. This ridge corresponds to the neck and shoulder area, which is often tense.

# The Reflexes Found on the Ball of the Feet

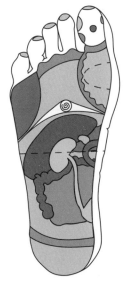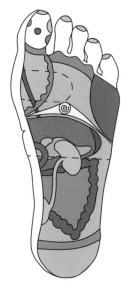

The area of the foot that runs from the bottom of the toes to the diaphragm line relates to the trunk and all the organs in this area, as well as the shoulder blades and shoulders. This relates to the top two areas, which are marked in pink in the accompanying illustration.

## The Lungs

The lungs supply every cell in the body with oxygen. Air is breathed in through the nose or mouth, warmed up in the nasal passage, then travels down the trachea, or windpipe. The windpipe branches into two bronchi, which take air into the lungs, and these divide into many more tubes called bronchioles. At the end of each bronchiole are small sacs called alveoli. An exchange of gases occurs in the walls of these tiny chambers.

## The Diaphragm

At the bottom of the chest below the lungs, there is a large muscle called the diaphragm. This muscle, which separates the abdomen from the chest, helps the ribs move in and out, squeezing and expanding the lungs. The diaphragm also increases abdominal pressure when the body needs to get rid of vomit, feces, and urine.

### Tip

The diaphragm line is between the yellow and green areas of the diagram on the previous page.

## The Chest

The chest consists of the ribs and the muscles in between, called the intercostals. It is the region of the thorax between the neck and the diaphragm in the front of the body.

## The Heart

The heart is approximately the size of your fist. It pumps blood around the body, beating more than 100,000 times a day. It consists of two halves, with two chambers (an atrium and a ventricle) in each half, and a valve that controls the blood flow between the two sides.

Deoxygenated blood enters the heart via the right atrium and travels into the right ventricle. Then the blood is pumped to the lungs via the pulmonary artery. Oxygenated blood from the lungs travels back to the heart via the pulmonary veins, entering the left atrium then the left ventricle through the aorta, and then it is pumped around the body.

### Tip

High levels of stress hormones in the bloodstream will cause the heart to beat faster. Breathing exercises and yoga can help calm the heartbeat.

## The Solar Plexus

Below the diaphragm line on the feet, there is an area that connects with the solar plexus and the nerves within it. This area contains a network of nerves in the autonomic (involuntary) nervous system that is responsible for regulating the organs. It is located between Zones 2 and 3 on both feet, beneath the diaphragm line.

## The Circulatory System

Arteries transport oxygenated blood around the body. Capillaries are smaller blood vessels through which blood passes to nourish the body, remove waste fluids, and remove deoxygenated blood. Capillaries flow into veins, which carry this deoxygenated blood back to the heart. Blood pressure is the pressure of blood that presses on the walls of the arteries. A perfect blood pressure reading is 120/80. Stress may cause blood pressure to rise, but blood pressure can vary throughout the day and from week to week. Reflexology can help treat high or low blood pressure.

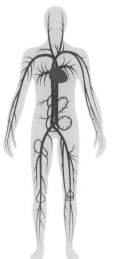

# The Reflexes Found on the Middle of the Foot

The middle of the foot corresponds to the central part of the body and organs found in this area.

## The Solar Plexus

Located in the stomach area, in front of the stomach wall, this is the area that is associated with "butterflies in the stomach." The solar plexus is a network of nerves, so reflexology that works on this area can be highly beneficial. Gently massaging this area brings a sense of emotional well-being as well as relaxation. This area can be tender if someone is experiencing a lot of emotional stress or is in constant pain.

## The Digestive System

A healthy digestive system is essential to good health and well-being. A dysfunctional digestive system not only prevents essential nutrients from being absorbed, but it can also make daily life unpleasant. Symptoms of a dysfunctional digestive system are:

- Diarrhea
- Constipation
- Pain
- Discomfort
- Bloating
- Burping
- Gas
- Reflux (or heartburn)

Reflexology can help return balance to a stressed digestive system. Many of us eat on the go, and a stressful daily routine can routinely cause digestive problems. Taking time out for reflexology can provide support for an overworked digestive system.

## The Liver

The liver, the largest organ in the body, is responsible for many functions, ranging from producing bile and cholesterol to breaking down toxic substances such as alcohol or medication into less harmful substances that the body can remove. This makes the liver the major detoxifying organ. It is able to store fats, sugars, and proteins until the body needs them, as well as process nutrients from the blood. The gallbladder stores the bile that the liver produces, releasing it into the small intestines, where it breaks down fat and fat-soluble vitamins so that the body can absorb them.

## The Stomach

Located on the left side of the body beneath the rib cage, the stomach is a stretchy muscular bag that breaks down food and releases gastric juices to enable digestion. It is usually approximately ten inches long but will expand to hold one quart of food.

## The Pancreas

The pancreas is a large organ that sits behind the stomach, mostly on the left side of the body. One task that this organ performs is helping to control blood sugar levels by producing the hormone insulin. The other part produces digestive enzymes, including protease to break down proteins, lipase to break down fat, and amylase to break down carbohydrates. These enzymes are released into the small intestine to continue the process of digestion once food has left the stomach.

## The Spleen

The spleen, which is part of the lymphatic system, is found on the left side of the body, behind the stomach and beneath the diaphragm. It produces lymphocytes and filters damaged red blood cells. It also filters the lymph (the fluid that contains white blood cells), which bathes the body's tissues, removing toxins and bacteria. The spleen also produces antibodies, thus making it an essential part of the immune system. Its reflex area is located two finger widths above the "waist line" on the left foot.

# The Waist Line

The waist line can be located below the notch on the side of the foot (see page 24), and it is found on the sole down to the heel area. It corresponds to the lower digestive system.

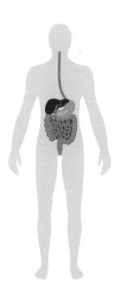

## The Small Intestine

The small intestine is approximately twenty-two feet long, and its function is to process food. The first section, the duodenum, is about one foot long. The digestive enzymes made by the pancreas are released into the duodenum. After the stomach has released its contents into the duodenum, these need to be neutralized to prevent the acidic contents from damaging the lining of the duodenum and causing ulcers. The second section of the small intestine is called the jejunum, and the last section is the ileum. This section, about twelve feet long, is where most nutrients are absorbed.

## The Ileocecal Valve

This valve is located between the small and large intestines. It prevents fecal matter from returning into the small intestine.

## The Appendix

The appendix is located at the beginning of the large intestine. The function of this organ is unknown, although it may serve as a reservoir for beneficial gut bacteria and some people believe it lubricates the colon. This organ is not absolutely necessary, so if it becomes infected or damaged in any way, it is often removed.

## The Large Intestine

Even though the large intestine is shorter than the small intestine, being just five feet in length, it is a wider tube than the small intestine. It's U-shaped and divided into four sections: the ascending colon, the transverse colon, the descending colon, and the sigmoid colon. The function of the large intestine is to absorb water and remove waste matter and mucus. Constipation is a common ailment of this section of the intestines, compounded by our modern diet and busy lifestyles.

## The Sigmoid Colon

This is the last section of the large intestine, before waste enters the rectum. It forms a loop of about fourteen to sixteen inches and resembles in shape the Greek letter sigma ($\Sigma$). Its function is to expel solid and gaseous waste from the gastrointestinal tract.

## The Urinary System

Also known as the renal system, this consists of the bladder, urethra, and kidneys. It produces, stores, and eliminates urine, the fluid waste excreted by the kidneys.

## The Kidneys

These organs are located in the back on either side of the spine, above the waist and underneath the rib cage. They are the body's main filtering organs, removing toxins and waste products from the blood. They also produce urine for excretion through the bladder. The kidneys regulate the balance of minerals and fluids in the body. Blood enters the kidneys through the medulla from the renal artery; it is filtered and then passes to the tubules, which are surrounded by tiny capillaries. These remove the useful chemicals and minerals to be transported back into the bloodstream via the renal vein. The waste that remains then passes via the urethra into the bladder. The kidneys are able to process about fifty gallons of blood a day.

## The Bladder

The bladder, located behind the pelvic bone, is a hollow muscular bag with a sphincter at the bottom that keeps fluid in the bladder until it's ready to empty. Urine then leaves the bladder through a tube called the urethra.

## The Adrenal Glands

These two small glands sit on top of the kidneys and are involved in many different functions. They produce hormones involved in vasoconstriction (constriction of blood vessels), muscle contraction, increased heart rate, increased breathing rate, and stress. They produce hormones that have an anti-inflammatory effect and are involved in sexual development, allergies, energy, and menopause. Stressful, busy lifestyles can put these glands under too much strain.

## The Spine

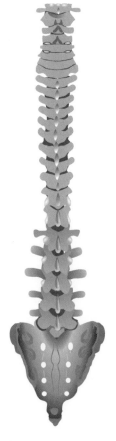

The spine consists of small bones, called vertebrae, that fit together to protect the spinal cord. This complex structure affects every function in the body. It needs to be both strong and flexible. Seven cervical vertebrae form the neck; twelve thoracic vertebrae make up the back; and five lumbar vertebrae form the lower back. Below these are the sacrum and coccyx, vertebrae that are fused together at the bottom of the spine.

The vertebrae act as protection for the spinal cord, which feeds the entire body with nerves. Messages to and from the brain travel along this cord, and it consciously and subconsciously coordinates all the functions of the body. Problems in the spine can cause problems in the organ or system related to the area of the spine that's affected. This reflex zone should be carefully and thoroughly worked on as it can affect the whole body.

Many people spend a substantial part of their day either at a desk or screen, or driving, encouraging a hunched and slouched position in the back, which can cause many aches and pains. Muscles spend a prolonged time in an unnatural position, which can lead to poor posture and neck and back ache.

## The Sciatic Nerve

The sciatic nerve runs from the buttocks down the leg to the base of the heel; when you work on this area in the foot, you're not working on a reflex point but the end of the nerve. If a disk or muscle presses on the nerve, pain can be felt down the leg and can cause discomfort whether sitting, walking, or exercising.

## Dermatomes and Myotomes

Dermatomes are areas on the skin, and myotomes are areas in muscle. Sensory neurons carry messages from our skin to the spinal cord and onward to the brain. If something touches our skin but we can't feel it, it shows that the nerves supplying the dermatome are either damaged or inflamed. This can also relate to a part of the spinal cord being damaged or inflamed. Myotomes function in a similar way, so if an area of muscle is paralyzed, the motor neurons in that spinal section may be inflamed or damaged.

If people have numb areas in their hands and feet, refer them to their general practitioner (GP) and/or a registered chiropractor.

# The Heel Area

The heel area of the foot corresponds to the reproductive system in both men and women.

## The Female Reproductive System

The female reproductive system consists of the uterus, two fallopian tubes, and two ovaries.

## The Uterus

The uterus, or womb, is where a baby grows, and it is situated at the top of the vagina, behind the bladder. It is held in place by a series of muscles and ligaments attached to the pelvic floor and the pelvis. It consists of a wall of thick muscle, which protects a growing embryo.

## The Fallopian Tubes

These tubes are responsible for propelling the egg that is released by the ovaries to the uterus by a series of wave-like movements, aided by tiny threadlike protrusions. There is one fallopian tube and one ovary on each side of the uterus.

## The Ovaries

Once a month, ovaries release a ripe egg that travels along the fallopian tubes into the uterus. The ovaries are also responsible for the production of estrogen. During menopause, in the later forties and early fifties, they eventually stop producing estrogen; however, a small amount is still made by the body from fat cells and the adrenal glands.

## The Male Reproductive System

The male reproductive system consists of two testes, the prostate gland, and the vas deferens, which is the tube through which semen and sperm pass.

## The Prostate Gland

This gland is located at the base of the bladder, at the first part of the urethra, and its secretions give sperm a fluid to swim in. Often as men age, the prostate can become swollen or inflamed, leading to the need to urinate frequently.

## The Testes

These two organs are found outside of the body to ensure they stay cool. They produce approximately fifty million sperm every day. The seminal vesicle then stores the mature sperm. The testes also produce the hormone testosterone, which gives men their male characteristics.

## Mucous Membranes

These membranes are found in the digestive, reproductive, and respiratory systems. They are linked by a reflex connection, so if one is affected, they can all be affected. Mucus is produced by the body to protect it from foreign invaders entering the bloodstream. The air we breathe in passes into the lungs, where a mucous lining catches foreign particles such as pollen and dust. The food we eat is also initially perceived by the body as foreign until it has been broken down by the mucous lining into recognizable molecules.

# The Overall Foot

There are some systems and elements of the body that correspond to areas all over the feet.

## The Lymphatic System

The lymphatic system consists of a network of vessels distributed throughout the body, and it is part of our immune system. It exists through the body and works closely with the circulatory system. Wherever you are working on the feet or hands, you will be working on the lymphatic system.

## The Skeletal System

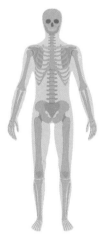

The skeleton exists to support the body and organs, and to help us move. There are 206 bones in the body, and these are separated into long bones, short bones, flat bones, and irregularly shaped bones. Bones have a hard exterior and a spongy interior, making them strong but light. Bones act as storage for calcium, which is needed for the blood to clot properly. If the system is too acidic, the body will release calcium reserves from the bones to neutralize this acidity in the blood. Reflex zones for the skeleton are found in many areas in the feet.

## The Muscular System

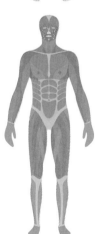

Muscles are grouped into skeletal muscles, which can be moved and are called "voluntary" muscles; and smooth muscles, also known as "involuntary" muscles, which ensure that our organs work while we sleep; and the cardiac muscle, which is also involuntary. Reflex zones for the muscular system are found in many areas of the feet.

## The Nervous System

This system consists of the spine, brain, and solar plexus, and every time reflexology is given, the whole of the nervous system is stimulated. The central nervous system includes the brain and spinal cord. The peripheral nervous system includes the autonomic (involuntary) nervous system. Working on the solar plexus reflex point will help relax the whole nervous system.

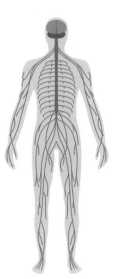

❊ ❊ ❊

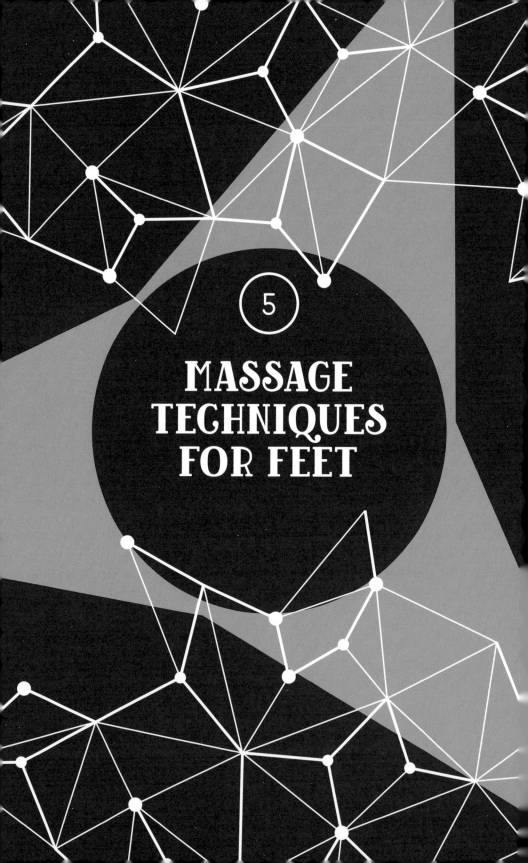

5

# MASSAGE TECHNIQUES FOR FEET

How you start a reflexology treatment will set the atmosphere for the rest of the session. After doing a few treatments, it will be easy to start establishing a routine. Make sure you have prepared the space where you are giving the treatment. Always have extra blankets within reach as sitting down for an hour can cause the body's temperature to drop. Whether you are working on your own feet or someone else's, you'll start each treatment from the toe end of the foot, gradually moving down as you progress.

## Finger Placement Technique

To perform reflexology properly, you will need to learn the correct way to use your thumb and index finger. On either the hands or the feet, you need to aim for a "caterpillar" movement with your thumb or index finger constantly moving forward.

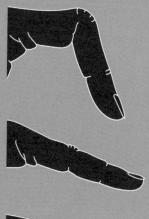

Use the ends of your fingers but not the tips, and ensure the movement is constantly moving forward in tiny steps, without sliding. If the skin is being pulled back, you're not moving forward.

As your fingers and thumbs become more used to working in this way, they will become stronger, and you will soon become accustomed to applying a consistent pressure. Some people prefer a lighter touch, whereas others like deep reflexology; if you are working on another person, your intuition will help you to get this right.

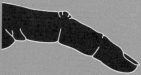

The correct finger positions.

Take a look at the sole of a foot and push the toes up and back, and you'll see a ligament that runs down the foot. Make sure to keep the foot relaxed enough that you can't see or feel this ligament, because working on a tense ligament will cause discomfort.

Never apply too much pressure, and be aware of any tender areas as your thumb or fingers work. The pressure needs to be firm enough not to tickle but not so firm that it hurts. Eventually you will learn a smooth and consistent technique. Remember to release the pressure between each tiny caterpillar step, and never slide the thumb or finger along the skin. Practice on your own hands, and as you become more experienced you will begin to feel tiny deposits that feel gritty. These are the blocked energy areas.

## Hands or Feet

The techniques in this chapter are described for the feet, but if you can't work on the feet due to injury, work on the hands instead. Here are the parts of the feet and legs and what parts of the hands and arms they correspond to. For more on massaging hands, see chapter 8.

| Foot and Leg | Hand and Arm |
| --- | --- |
| Sole of foot | Palm of hand |
| Top of foot | Back of hand |
| Big toe | Thumb |
| Small toes | Fingers |
| Ankle | Wrist |
| Calf | Forearm (inner) |
| Shin | Forearm (outer) |
| Knee | Elbow |
| Thigh | Upper arm |
| Hip | Shoulder |

# Massage Techniques

As you experiment and become more confident in giving a reflexology treatment, you will discover techniques that help with relaxation. One of the best ways to find out what really works is to have a treatment yourself. Alternatively, ask friends to let you practice on them and to give you feedback about what is the most effective.

## Making a Connection

Here is a very simple massage routine you can do to start to familiarize yourself with reflexology massage and making a connection with the people you treat:

- Have the person lie down on their back. Place the palms of your hands on the soles of both feet to establish a connection with your recipient, and hold them there for twenty to thirty seconds.
- Then place your hands under and around the back of the person's heels, gently but firmly holding the heels in your hands. As you lean back a little, raise the legs slightly and slowly pull toward yourself to stretch the legs. Relax for ten seconds and then repeat, until you feel the person is beginning to relax.
- Keeping contact and using the same gentle grip, put the person's legs back down and rock them from side to side. Repeat this up to five times to release tension in the person's back.

## Warming Up

Before you begin working on the different reflex areas, you will need to warm up the person's feet with a basic massage. What follows is a ten-step sequence to do just that. Massage each foot at each step before progressing to the next step. Once you have worked on one foot, wrap it in a towel to keep it warm as you work on the other foot.

## Warm-Up Step One

Place your left hand under the right heel, your right hand over the foot, and your thumb under the right foot (thumb pointing toward little toe). Gently rotate the ankle in one direction and then in the other direction several times to loosen the joint.

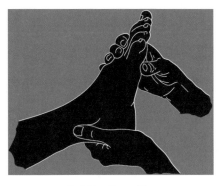

Rotating the ankle.

## Warm-Up Step Two

Using both hands, rotate the ankles in opposite directions, gently squeezing them. Do this up to ten times.

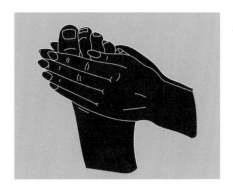

Rotating the upper and lower areas of the foot.

## Warm-Up Step Three

Place your right hand on top of the left foot. Make a fist with your left hand and put it in the ball of the foot. Gently push with the fist, as you slowly rotate it back and forth. Do this several times.

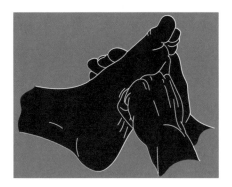

Rotating the sole of the foot.

## Warm-Up Step Four

Place both of your thumbs under the foot and all your fingers on top of the foot. Starting at the bottom of the foot, move your fingers using the caterpillar technique across the top of the foot.

Work the fingers toward each other without meeting. Repeat this, each time moving up the foot. Return to the starting position and do it again.

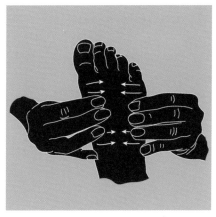

Massaging the sides of the foot.

## Warm-Up Step Five

Hold the heel of the foot with the left hand. With the fingers of the right hand starting at the top of the foot just below the toes, use a gentle caterpillar movement to massage downward, toward the ankle. Return to the starting position and do this several times more.

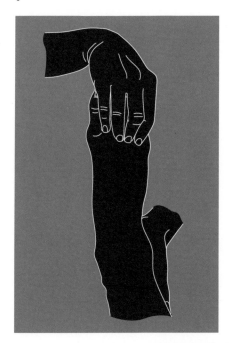
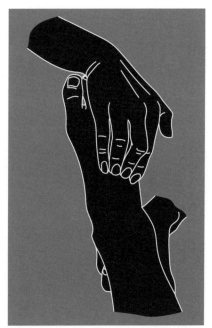

Massaging the top of the foot.

## Warm-Up Step Six

Using the caterpillar technique, move your thumbs across the bottom of foot with each thumb going in the opposite direction to the other. Do this up and down the length of the foot several times.

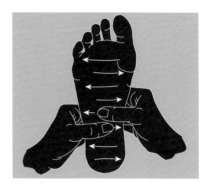

Massaging the sides of the foot.

## Warm-Up Step Seven

With one hand, cup the heel of the foot. Make a fist with the other hand and gently apply pressure as you move down the foot. Do this several times.

## Warm-Up Step Eight

Gently pull each toe to stretch it. Rub down the front of the toe and then rotate it right and left.

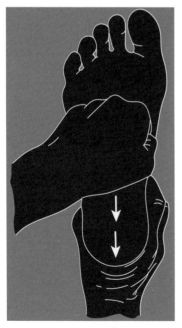

Massaging the sole of the foot.

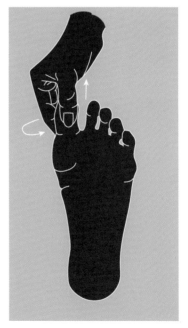

Stretching the toes.

## Warm-Up Step Nine

Place your palms on each side of the foot and slide your hands up and down the sides of the foot.

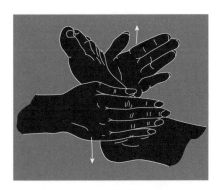

Massaging the sides of the foot.

## Warm-Up Step Ten

Place one hand under the Achilles tendon at the back of the ankle and hold the top of the foot with the other hand. Apply pressure on the foot in order to stretch it. Hold for a few seconds. Then move the top hand under the top of the foot and gently apply pressure to stretch the Achilles tendon.

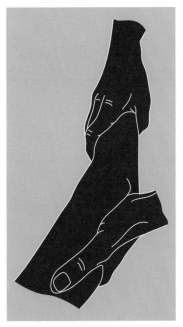
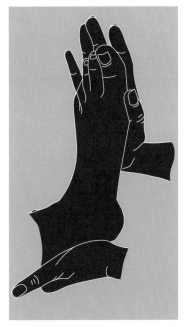

Stretching the Achilles tendon.

❄ ❄ ❄

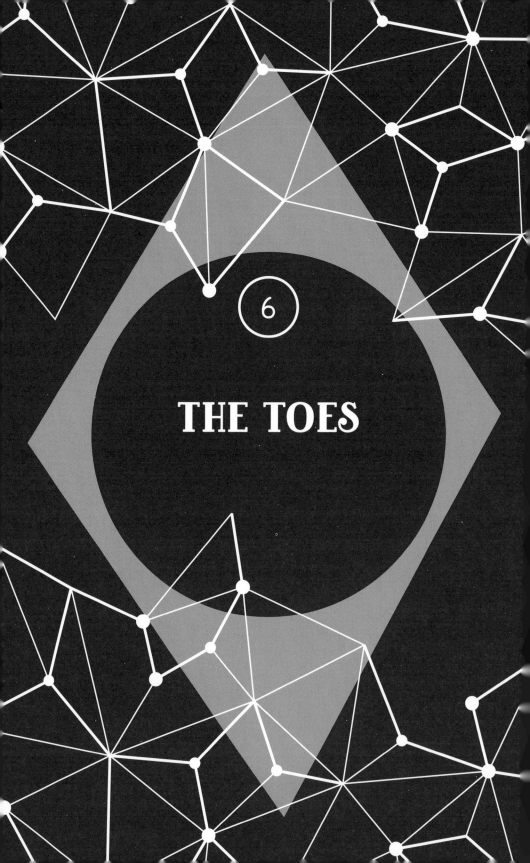

# 6

# THE TOES

After you have warmed up one foot and the other foot with a gentle massage, such as the one described in chapter 5, you can go on to work with the reflex areas. This chapter gives details on massage techniques you can use to treat ailments in different reflex areas of the toes. These areas correspond to the neck, head, and shoulders. For more details on this, refer back to chapters 2, 3, and 4.

## The Sinuses, Neck, Head, and Shoulders

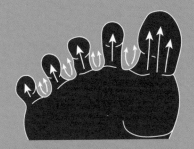

Some people suffer from stress headaches, or blocked and infected sinuses. Children can sometimes suffer from head and neck pain due to stress. Active children who spend a lot of time after school involved in competitive sports can suffer from tight shoulders and experience neck pain. People who suffer from migraines can benefit from work on the neck, head, and shoulders, as well as anyone finding it difficult to relax and drop off to sleep at night.

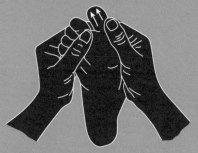

### Treatment

You need to work on the toes for these areas of the body, so hold the right foot with your left hand and "caterpillar walk" up the big toe with your right thumb. Repeat four or five times going from the base to the top, covering the whole area. Use the right index finger to walk up the side of the next toe, and then use the thumb to walk up the middle of that toe. Repeat this process until you reach the

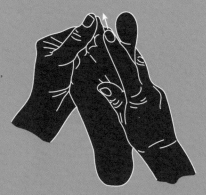

Treating the sinuses, neck, head, and shoulders.

little toe, then change hands and work your way up the middle of the small toe with your left thumb. Then change to your left index finger and work your way up the side of the toe. Repeat the process again, moving from the small toe to the big one.

## The Eyes and Ears

Babies and children who suffer from earache can benefit from very gentle work on these areas, as can older people who get frequent ear infections. Many people may also complain of hay fever that affects the eyes or causes congestion in the ears. Migraine can also be associated with the eyes, and head colds can affect both eyes and ears. Tired eyes may occur due to overuse of screens, in both younger people and office workers, and in those who are under a lot of pressure

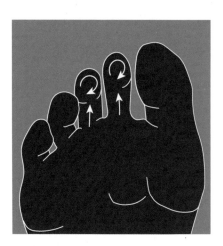
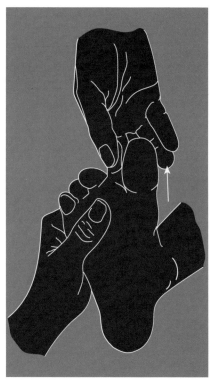

Treating the eyes and ears.

at work. For older people who cannot read as regularly as they once did, due to deterioration of vision, or who have hearing loss or tinnitus, work on these reflexes.

## Treatment

Hold the right foot with your left hand and pull the second toe, rotating the thumb around the fleshy part of the toe. Repeat on the next toe (the second toe along from the big toe). This circular movement is used on the toes but not on any other part of the foot.

# The Neck and Thyroid

Common complaints in these areas can be living with an over- or underactive thyroid, or an abnormality in the production of the thyroid hormones. Neck issues can range from physical injuries, such as whiplash resulting from a car accident or injury when participating in a sport, to tension throughout the back, neck, and head that is referring pain to this area. Poor posture and prolonged time either at a desk or driving a car can contribute to neck issues. When a high level of neck tension exists, it is important to use good posture, which means standing tall with a neutral spine, and with the shoulders kept down and held back, avoiding slouching where the shoulders fall forward.

## Treatment

Hold the right foot in your left hand and work your right thumb across the base of the first three toes, using a caterpillar movement from the base of the big toe to the base of the third toe. Do this twice.

Then make a fist with your left hand and fit it onto the ball of the right foot. On the top of the foot, walk across the foot from the base of the first three toes. Do this with both your right index finger and second finger working together, starting with the big toe. Do this twice.

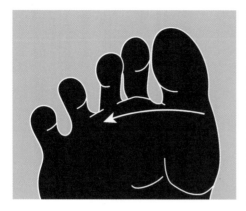
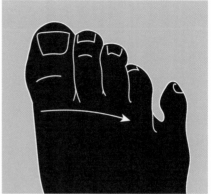
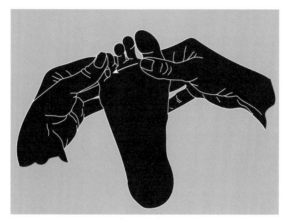
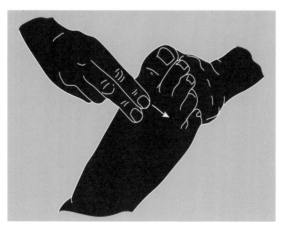

Treating the neck and thyroid.

# The Face

Many people hold tension in the muscles of their face, whether it is in the forehead, the miniscule muscles around the eyes, the cheeks, or the muscles that surround the jawbone. Others may present with an injury to the face, such as a burn or a cut. Skin problems are extremely common, and can range from acne to rosacea, eczema, and irregular pigmentation. Overexposure to the sun may result in skin cancer.

## Treatment

Make a fist with your left hand to keep the ball of the foot steady, and then use your right index finger to work across the large toe, just below the nail bed. Do this twice.

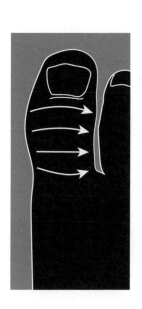 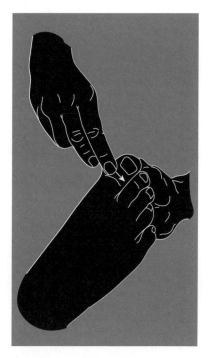

Treating the face.

❋ ❋ ❋

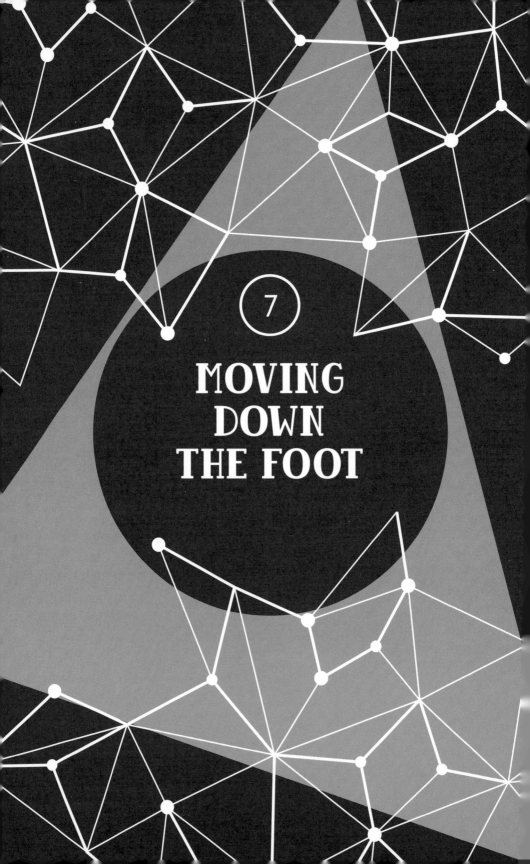

# 7

# MOVING
# DOWN
# THE FOOT

After you've addressed the toes of one foot and then the other foot, you can move down the foot to the reflex areas that correspond to the trunk of the body as well as the limbs. For more details on these areas, refer back to chapters 2, 3, and 4.

## The Chest

Issues that occur in the chest may arise due to infection. Physical trauma to the chest can also occur due to injury, such as cracked ribs or other broken bones resulting from participation in sports or from car crashes. Loss of height due to aging can compress ribs and cause pain in this area. Stress can also lead to issues in this area, especially as it can trigger asthma attacks. Chest pain can also be caused by a more serious underlying problem. Anyone presenting with chest pain should be encouraged to make an appointment with their general practitioner (GP).

### Treatment

Hold the foot steady in one hand and use the index finger of the other hand to make a caterpillar movement down from the toes, across the diaphragm area.

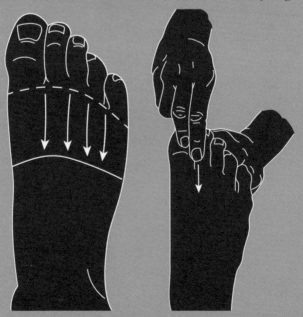

Treating the chest.

# The Liver and Gallbladder

Gallstones are crystallized fatty deposits, usually made from cholesterol that forms in the gallbladder, which is a small pear-shaped organ on the right side of the abdomen, just beneath the liver. If these stones become trapped in an opening inside the gallbladder, they can trigger intense stomach pain. Jaundice, or yellow-tinted skin, may be a sign of a block or stone in the common bile duct, which leads from the gallbladder to the small intestine.

There are over 100 different types of liver disease. Some of the most common types include alcohol-related liver disease, hepatitis, and primary biliary cirrhosis, which may be caused by a problem with the immune system. Advise people with liver or alcohol issues to drink plenty of water, and be aware that those who are struggling with alcoholism may also have underlying anxiety issues.

## Treatment

Hold the right foot in your left hand and work the area from the diaphragm line to the waist line, at the angle shown in the accompanying illustrations. Ninety percent of the liver's reflex area is on the right foot.

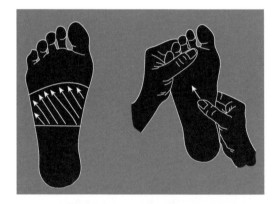

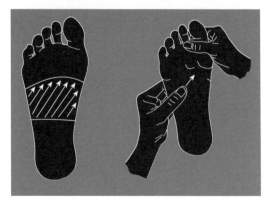

Treating the liver and gallbladder.

# The Lungs, Chest, Heart, and Shoulders

The most common lung diseases include asthma, inflammation of the bronchial tubes known as bronchitis, COPD (chronic obstructive pulmonary disease), cancer, and infection (pneumonia). If an infection or a disease isn't treated, it can worsen quickly, so medical advice should be sought.

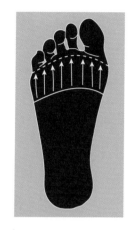

Heart disease generally refers to conditions that involve narrowed or blocked blood vessels that can lead to a heart attack or atrial fibrillation.

Shoulders can be affected by arthritis, torn cartilage, swollen tendons, pinched nerves, broken bones, and "frozen shoulder," which affects the shoulder joint and involves pain and stiffness. A very busy lifestyle with a high level of stress, such as going through divorce or moving, can also lead to a buildup of tension in the shoulders.

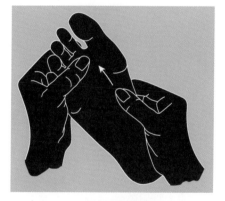

## Treatment

Take the right foot in your left hand and place your thumb on the upper part of the diaphragm area. Then, with your right thumb, move up to the toes using a caterpillar movement. Change hands and repeat the movement.

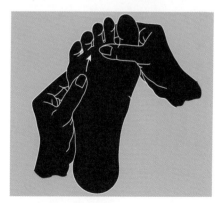

Treating the lungs, chest, heart, and shoulders.

# The Stomach, Pancreas, and Spleen

Stomach issues can sometimes be caused by stress or diet, and these can range from cramps to diarrhea and constipation. Abdominal pain can be caused by irritable bowel syndrome (IBS); if it is severe, people should be referred to their doctor. Many people don't eat conventional meals seated at a table; instead, they eat on the go, often rushing meals, eating ready-made food that is lacking in basic nutrients, and sometimes skipping meals. When stress is constantly present, along with a poor diet and too much alcohol, the stomach will often suffer.

The most common disorder of the pancreas is known as pancreatitis. With this condition, the pancreas becomes inflamed.

The spleen is a fist-sized organ in the upper left side of the abdomen, next to the stomach and behind the left ribs. If it's not working properly, this can lead to anemia and increased risk of infection. A ruptured spleen that has burst due to an injury, such as a car accident, can be removed. We can survive without the spleen.

## Treatment

Hold the left foot with your right hand, cradling the heel from below. Walk your other hand down the whole area from the diaphragm line to the waist line.

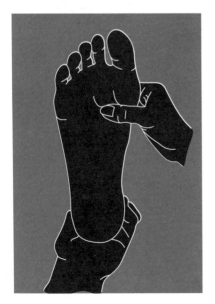 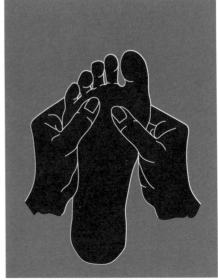

Treating the stomach, pancreas, and spleen.

# The Ileocecal Valve, Small and Large Intestines, and Sigmoid Colon

When the ileocecal valve isn't working, it can cause many symptoms, from shoulder pain to dizziness to fever. Small intestine problems can range from celiac disease (sensitivity to gluten) to Crohn's and other inflammatory bowel diseases (IBDs), cancer, and ulcers. Issues with the large intestine can include colorectal cancer, colonic polyps (extra tissue growths in the colon), ulcers, inflammation, and irritable bowel syndrome (IBS). Just as with some stomach issues, modern-day living with high levels of stress, long working hours, and fast food can affect the functioning of the intestines. The sigmoid colon is the last section of the bowel that attaches to the rectum. Problems in this area may present as abdominal pain, nausea, loss of appetite, diarrhea, or constipation.

## Treatment

Cradle the right heel in your right hand and use your thumb to rub firmly across the foot from the center of the sole to the outside edge of the foot. Next, work the area from the waist line downward using your left thumb, working from one side of the foot to the other. Then change hands and use your left thumb to work across the area, down to the end.

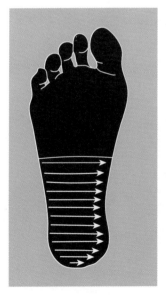

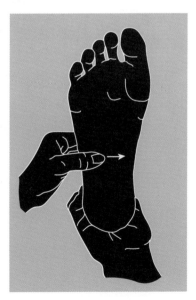

Treating the ileocecal valve, small intestine, and large intestine.

Treating the sigmoid colon.

# The Spine, Hips, and Pelvic Area

A slipped or herniated disk between the vertebrae of the spine can be extremely painful, and it can limit movement. Osteoarthritis can wear down the cartilage between the vertebrae. Pressure on the sciatic nerve (sciatica) can also be debilitating. Spinal cord injury can lead to partial paralysis. A common complaint among pregnant women is hip and pelvic pain. Sports injuries, as well as pelvic floor issues, can also affect the hips and pelvis.

## Treatment

Use your left hand to support the right foot, about halfway down on the outside edge. Work your thumb up the inside of the foot, along the arch, bringing your fingers around to the front of the foot. Start at the bottom and work up to the top of the big toe, then return to the beginning. Do this twice.

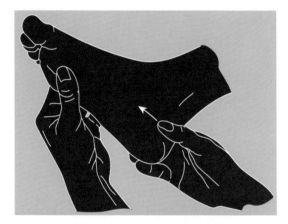

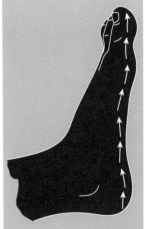

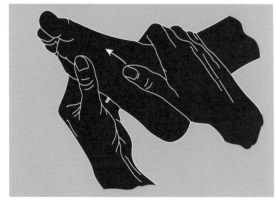

Treating the spine, hips, and pelvic area.

# The Kidneys, Bladder, and Adrenal Glands

Abnormality of the kidneys is referred to as kidney disease; when it is labeled "chronic," it means the condition lingers and may not become completely cured, though this doesn't necessarily mean the condition is severe. Kidney disease is very common, but fewer than one in ten people with kidney disease develop failure of the kidney that would require dialysis or a transplant.

A common condition of the bladder, especially in women, is cystitis. With age, bladder problems can become more common, but the discomfort they cause can be eased with reflexology. Loss of bladder control, frequent need to urinate, and leaking urine are symptoms of lower urinary tract problems. Often, women will suffer some or all of these after giving birth. Encourage people with bladder issues to drink plenty of water every day. Children can suffer from bed-wetting, especially if they are experiencing stress, such as starting a new grade in school, moving, or when a new sibling is due.

Adrenal glands produce hormones that help regulate metabolism, the immune system, blood pressure, and stress.

## Treatment

The bladder reflex is a slightly puffy area along the reflex of the spine just where the arch of the foot begins. With your left hand, hold the right foot and use your right thumb to move from the bladder reflex area and along the ligament of the foot without pressing too hard on the ligament itself. Make sure the foot isn't stretched too much to avoid hurting the sensitive ligament.

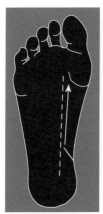 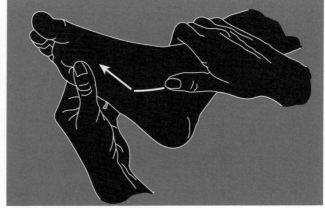

Treating the kidneys, bladder, and adrenal glands.

Stop when you are a couple of finger widths from the diaphragm. Return to the bladder reflex point and do this twice more, then rotate the adrenal reflex point several times to finish.

# The Reproductive System

Women can suffer from many issues related to the reproductive system throughout their lives, especially concerning their monthly periods, pregnancy, and menopause.

Endometriosis occurs when the lining of the womb grows in other areas, such as on the ovaries, on the bowels, or on the bladder. Cancer can also affect the cervix, ovaries, uterus, vagina, and vulva. Polycystic ovary syndrome (PCOS) results when the ovaries produce more male hormones than normal, causing cysts to develop on the ovaries. Sexual violence can also lead to trauma of the reproductive system, as well as have complex emotional and psychological repercussions.

In men, reproductive health problems can include impotence, testicular disorders, and prostate cancer.

## Treatment

Hold the right foot in your right hand and move your left thumb from the back of the outside of the heel to the anklebone. Do this twice. Now change hands so that you are holding the right foot with your left hand and work your right thumb from the tip of the heel on the inside of the foot to the anklebone. Repeat the procedure twice.

Now put both thumbs onto the sole of the right foot; then, with the first two fingers of both hands, work on the top of the foot, starting at each anklebone and working around the ankle until your fingers meet in the middle. Do this twice.

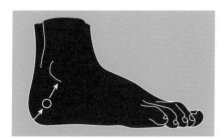

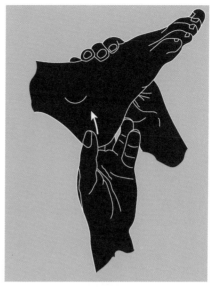

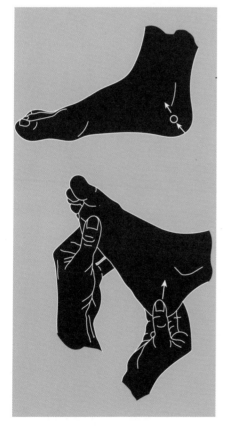

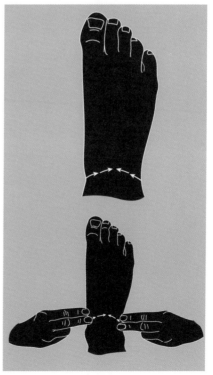

Treating the reproductive system.

# The Coccyx

Pain in and around this bony structure at the bottom of the spine can be caused by trauma such as falling, prolonged sitting, degeneration of the joint, and childbirth. During the end of pregnancy, the coccyx becomes more flexible to allow it to bend and give way during birth. Sometimes, childbirth causes the muscles and ligaments around the coccyx to overstretch. A few sports, such as cycling and rowing—where the person continually leans forward, stretching the base of the spine—may lead to coccyx pain. Poor posture, as well as being overweight or underweight, can lead to discomfort. Sitting in an awkward position, such as at a desk all day or driving a car for long periods of time, can also put too much pressure on the coccyx. Thin people who spend a lot of time sitting in front of computers tend to become very sore in this area, due to the pressure on the tail end of the spine.

## Treatment

Support the heel of the right foot with your left hand and hold the upper part of the foot with your right hand. Use your fingers on your left hand to work across the inside of the heel.

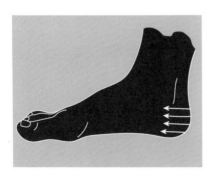
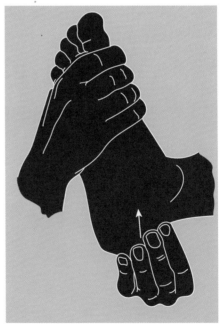

Treating the coccyx.

# The Hips and Pelvis

Many forms of arthritis and related conditions that affect the joints, muscles, or bones can cause hip problems like pain, stiffness, and swelling. The sciatic nerve runs from the lower part of the spinal cord through the buttock and down the back of the leg to the foot. Sciatica may be felt as a sharp or burning pain that radiates from the hip. Hip pain can also be caused by overuse or sports injuries.

## Treatment

Take the right foot in your right hand and cradle the person's heel. Use the four fingers of your right hand to work across the outside of the heel while supporting the upper part of the foot with your left hand.

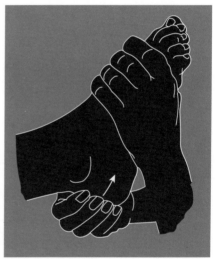

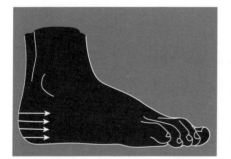

Treating the hips and pelvis.

# The Shoulders

Shoulder pain can be a symptom of an underlying condition and can manifest in long-term pain and stiffness, due to arthritis or frozen shoulder. If the pain is worse while using the arm, it may be due to tendonitis. Sudden intense pain that prevents the person moving an arm could be due to a dislocated shoulder, broken bone, or torn or ruptured tendon. If shoulder pain doesn't improve after two weeks, the person should seek advice from a doctor.

## Treatment

Supporting the right foot with your right fist, use your left index and middle fingers in a caterpillar movement across from the outside of two toe widths. Continue working downward to the diaphragm line, and do this twice more.

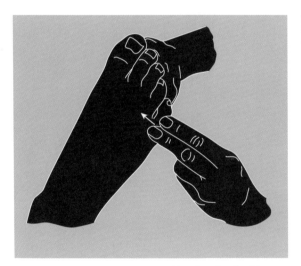 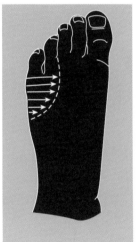

Treating the shoulders.

# The Arms, Knees, and Elbows

Arm and elbow pain is not usually a sign of
a serious underlying condition. For athletes
suffering from tennis elbow (tendonitis), a bag
of frozen peas wrapped in a towel and placed
on the area can help. The arm should be
raised if it's swollen. Sprains and strains may
cause bruising, swelling, tenderness, and pain.

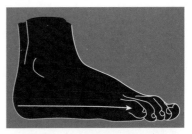

Knee pain can be a symptom of many
different conditions, including sprains
and strains, tendonitis, cartilage damage,
Osgood-Schlatter disease (suffered by
teenagers and young adults as their knees
are growing), and a dislocated kneecap. If
the knee is hot and red, with sudden attacks
of very bad pain, it could be due to gout,
which requires medical attention.

## Treatment

Hold the right foot with your right hand,
and use your left thumb to work up the
outside of the foot, starting at the heel and
finishing at the base of the little toe. Do
this once more.

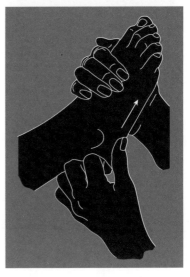

Treating the arms, knees, and elbows.

# Coming to the End of the Treatment

Finish with some gentle relaxation techniques. Sandwich the foot in both hands
and hold it still for thirty seconds, then cover the foot with a towel to keep
it warm. Repeat the treatment on the left foot. When you have finished the
treatment, perform a gentle, smooth massage on both feet. If you are working
with a client, place the palm of your right hand on the sole of the person's left
foot and the palm of your left hand on the sole of the right foot. Hold your
hands in place for a minute while the person slowly centers him- or herself.
Offer a drink of water and then wash your hands.

✳ ✳ ✳

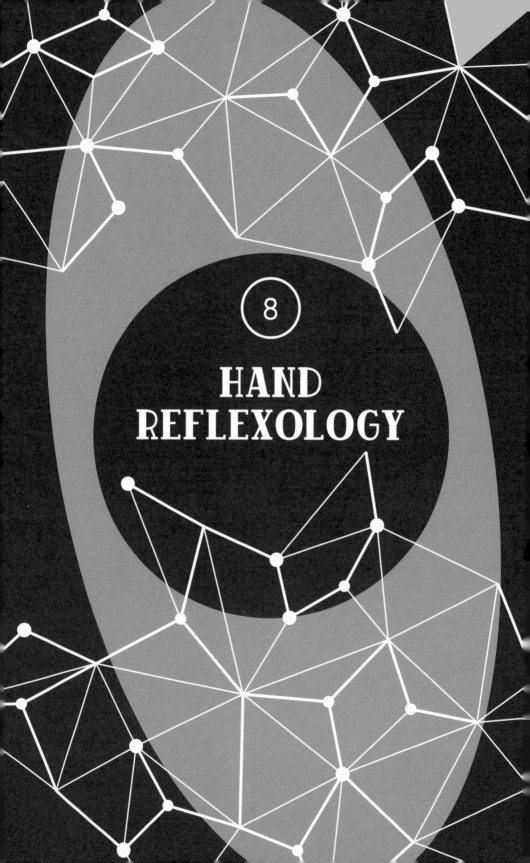

8

# HAND
# REFLEXOLOGY

Sometimes it's easier to do reflexology on the hands than on the feet, especially if the person you are working with has a problem with their feet, but do a scan of the hands before you make a decision. Avoid any areas of the hands where there is broken skin, eczema, psoriasis, warts, or a fungal infection. Hand reflexology is also something you can practice on yourself, anytime, anywhere.

The anatomy of the hands is very different from that of the feet. Almost half of the length of the hand is taken up by fingers, whereas the toes are only about one-sixth of the length of the feet. This means that reflexes below the shoulder line are more compressed on the hands, whereas reflexes above the shoulder line are more compressed on the feet. Potentially, this makes treating neck and shoulder issues much easier on the hands. As with foot reflexology, the palm side of your hand contains a lot more reflex points than the dorsal side. If you are working on hands and you feel something on a reflex point, check the hand map and see which area it is connected to.

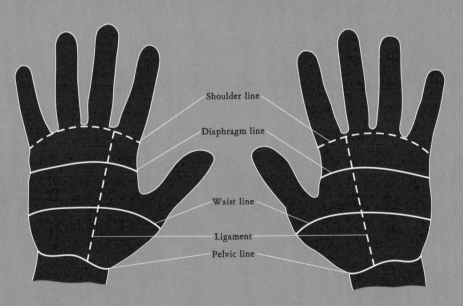

Shoulder line

Diaphragm line

Waist line

Ligament

Pelvic line

The divisions of the hands.

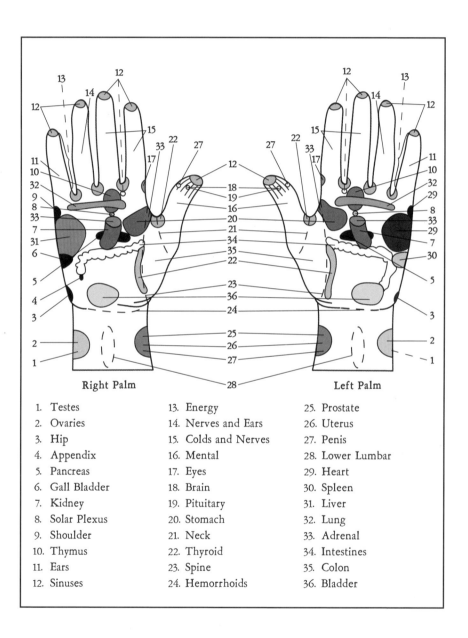

Right Palm

Left Palm

| | | |
|---|---|---|
| 1. Testes | 13. Energy | 25. Prostate |
| 2. Ovaries | 14. Nerves and Ears | 26. Uterus |
| 3. Hip | 15. Colds and Nerves | 27. Penis |
| 4. Appendix | 16. Mental | 28. Lower Lumbar |
| 5. Pancreas | 17. Eyes | 29. Heart |
| 6. Gall Bladder | 18. Brain | 30. Spleen |
| 7. Kidney | 19. Pituitary | 31. Liver |
| 8. Solar Plexus | 20. Stomach | 32. Lung |
| 9. Shoulder | 21. Neck | 33. Adrenal |
| 10. Thymus | 22. Thyroid | 34. Intestines |
| 11. Ears | 23. Spine | 35. Colon |
| 12. Sinuses | 24. Hemorrhoids | 36. Bladder |

# Benefits of Hand Reflexology

Hand reflexology can boost circulation, especially for those who suffer from Raynaud's disease, which makes the fingers numb and cold in response to cold temperatures. It can also provide pain relief from chronic problems such as arthritis or repetitive strain issues. Additionally, it may help increase flexibility in the joints, especially for those with rheumatoid arthritis. Most commonly, hand reflexology may provide relief from headaches and back pain, sinus and breathing problems, stress, anxiety, and irritable bowel syndrome (IBS). In general, it is also incredibly soothing and relaxing.

You might detect "crunchy" areas in the hands or fingers, which indicate blockages in the flow of energy somewhere in the body. Working on these areas will ease pain, allow the blood to clear toxins more easily, and promote the body's natural healing ability. Some people have adhesions in their body, which are fibrous tissues that are like scar tissue, and these can be eased by hand reflexology.

Working on the hands can be very calming and relaxing. When you are calmer and more relaxed, you are much more likely to let go of tension you may be holding in your muscles. As you enjoy the hand massage, hormones are released that increase your sense of happiness and well-being. If, by the end of a treatment, you are feeling calmer, happier, and more relaxed, you are more likely to benefit, both physically and emotionally.

# Five-Minute Practice

Here are some simple steps to help you make a start with hand reflexology. Once you feel comfortable doing this on yourself, you can try it on others.

- Relax the hand with deep, wide movements of your thumb sweeping across the palm, creating a semicircle as you work from the center outward. Spend a few seconds deeply massaging the area at the base of the thumb. Use small circular movements to then gently work downward in a line from each of the knuckles to the wrist, ensuring you don't press too hard.
- Wrap your whole hand around a finger and gently rub the joint. Then rotate the whole finger, and squeeze along the finger up to the tip.
- Pinch the end of each finger and hold the pressure for a couple of seconds before gently swiping away. Look at the map of the zones of the

hands to see which end point relates to which body part (each tip of each finger is different).

- Apply gentle pressure in small circles all over the back and front of the hand, working in toward the wrist.
- Make a fist with the hand you're working on, hold it with the other hand, and gently rotate the wrist joint first one way then the other.
- Repeat the whole massage on the other hand.

Once these techniques feel comfortable, try them on someone else. Start by placing one of your hands on top of the other person's hand and one below, as that will make the initial contact. Let them talk about any problems or issues they may be having. Often, this alone can help people let go of some of their burdens. After you have worked on specific areas, stretch the hand by gently holding the little finger and thumb and slowly pulling all the fingers apart. Finish with holding the person's whole hand in both of your hands again before you slowly detach yourself from the hand by sliding your hands away.

# Taking Hand Reflexology to the Next Level

- Start by gently massaging the inner side of the right wrist by sweeping your thumb in an outward motion.
- Do the same with the left wrist.
- Now put your thumb in the center of the palm and work toward the upper part of the outside of the hand. Do this again, traveling to the middle part of the side of the hand, then once again, aiming for the lower part of the side of the hand.
- Put your thumb back in the middle of the hand and work your way to the upper part of the other edge of the hand, then the middle part of the edge, then the lower part.
- Do the same for the other hand.
- Now do the same for the back of one hand, and then repeat the action on the other hand.
- Gently waggle each finger in turn, without pulling the fingers too much. Slowly massage each finger in turn, concentrating on the top side and underside of each finger, and then do it again focusing on the sides of each finger.

- Do the same with the fingers of the other hand.
- Now massage the thumb, working from the tip to the base, first on the top and underside of the thumb, then on the lateral sides.
- Do the same with the other thumb.

When you have finished, wash your hands and either have a drink of water or pour the person you're working with a drink of water. The water will help to clear the gases that occur due to the cleansing effect of the reflexology that sets off the process of removing toxins from the body.

* * *

# Another Form of Hand Reflexology

There is an older method of hand treatment that is somewhat different from the system outlined above, because it's based on palmistry. Unlike modern reflexology, palmistry has been around for more than 5,000 years, although the idea is much the same as for standard reflexology, in that you massage various areas of the hand to improve a health problem or to ease an emotional one. The beauty of this type of hand reflexology is that it is easy to do it on your own hands, but of course, you can use the technique on the hands of others, and because it is so gentle and noninvasive, you can even use the technique on children.

As it happens, seldom do amateur or professional reflexologist working on the hands, but palmists often use the method to help their clients, and so it's used much more frequently than the standard form of hand reflexology. This proves that there is room for more than one technique in this world.

The condition of our hands reflects our state of mind at any one time, and it also links to our character and talents, our faults and our destiny. So a reflexology treatment on the hands can help in many different ways in addition to improving one's health.

A palmist's "Map of the Hand" (see page 86) uses the planetary names for the various areas of the hands, but this isn't hard to understand, as all you need to do is check the illustration. The fingers are also easy to understand, and they work like this:

- The Jupiter finger is the index, or first, finger.
- The Saturn finger is the middle finger.

- The Apollo finger is the ring, or third, finger.
- The Mercury finger is the little finger.
- The thumb isn't associated with any planet.

# Fingernails

It is worth checking the fingernails, because nails take around eight months to grow from root to tip, so they show what has happened to the subject in recent months. For instance, when someone starts chemotherapy, a deep trench can form across the thumbnail. This kind of deep lateral groove comes about when something intensely toxic enters the bloodstream—such as the toxins found in chemotherapy.

There are other grooves, dents, and pits that show up when serious matters arise, but for the purposes of this book, it is only worth knowing that lateral dents show some kind of shock to the system. This could result from a bout of flu; dental treatment; a fall, especially if a bone gets broken; or even a badly stomach upset. Grooves show up when someone drinks too much caffeine or is going through some kind of traumatic event.

Pale nails indicate poor circulation or anemia, while blue or mauve ones can indicate a problem related to the arteries or the heart. Yellow nails talk of jaundice, while nails with white and brownish banding suggest kidney disease, liver disease, diabetes, alcoholism, or even HIV.

If the moons (the white arcs at the base of the nail) suddenly get larger, especially on the thumb and Jupiter (index) finger, there may be heart disease, liver problems, lung problems, or a host of other unpleasant ailments.

Grooves that run down the nails are very common, particularly among older people, especially if they have arthritis.

A problem with the head, neck, and spine will show up as a single longitudinal groove or ridge on the thumb and Jupiter fingernails. A problem with the bones, ligaments, and tendons surrounding the chest, shoulders, and pelvis will appear as a groove or ridge on the Saturn (middle) fingernails. A problem with the hips, elbows, and thighs shows up as grooves or ridges on the Apollo (ring) fingernails, while problems with the hands, feet, wrists, and ankles show up as grooves or ridges running down the Mercury (little) fingernails.

White spots on the nails often turn up in the spring because the person hasn't spent much time in the sun. It is worth taking a vitamin D and calcium supplement when these show up.

"Watch-glass nails" are called this because they become convex, rise from their beds and look like old-fashioned watch-glasses. These were well known to old-time doctors, because they are a classic sign of tuberculosis, but they are more likely to be linked to lung cancer these days.

## Fingers and Fingertips

Fatigue shows up as vertical creases that run down the inner sides of the fingers. More serious problems, such as insomnia, can be shown by lateral lines, but these also suggest that the person is being held back by other people in some way. It may take much more than a hand massage to cure these problems, but reflexology might help someone cope with them.

Lines across the fingertips show temporary hormonal problems, but if the fingerprints are almost obliterated, it can be due to serious eye problems.

Gently feel around the fingers to see if there are any cold spots, as they can indicate circulation problems. A gentle finger massage can be help circulation.

The upper palm area that lies directly below the fingers relates to the heart, lungs, and breasts. It is a good area to massage if you have a cold or feel a bit off.

## The Jupiter Finger

If you have a headache or feel sluggish, you can benefit from rubbing this finger. This is also useful if others are trying to put you down or push ahead of you in your career.

## The Saturn Finger

Saturn relates to bones, skin, and hearing, so any of these problems might benefit from treating this finger. If you are worried about your job or financial security, massage this finger. If you are engaged in agriculture or horticulture and need to give your career or hobby a boost, give this finger a rub.

## The Apollo Finger

This finger concerns the spine, heart, chest, and eyes. If you are struggling with a creative project, planning a building or decorating one, or doing something artistic or musical, give this finger a good massage.

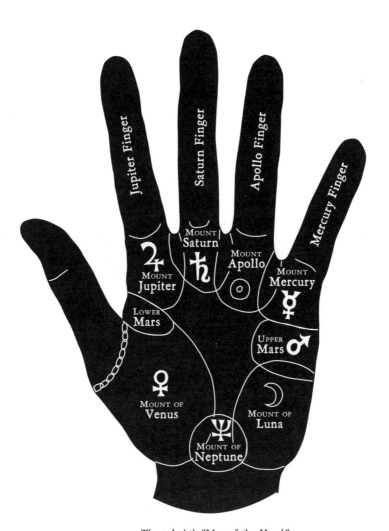

The palmist's "Map of the Hand."

## The Mercury Finger

This finger concerns communication, so if you have a sore throat or don't feel that you can speak clearly enough, or if you struggle to express yourself in writing, give this finger a rub. It also relates to the shoulders, arms, wrists, and hands, so arthritis in these areas might benefit from a massage here.

## The Thumb

This can relate to the head, neck, throat, and upper spine, so massage the thumb when these body areas are bothering you. The ball of the thumb relates to willpower, so if you need to have faith in yourself and to make something happen, rub this area. The lower joint of the thumb relates to logic and common sense, so if yours seems to be deserting you, give this area a good massage.

## The Mount of Jupiter

This area can relate to fatigue and some glandular problems, but also headaches due to fatigue. Lines here can refer to ambition, friendship, love, and luck, so give this area a massage for all round good fortune. This mount is also concerned with teaching and studying, so if these matters are important to you, give this mount some reflexology.

## The Mount of Saturn

The mount of Saturn is concerned with security, money, a decent job, respectability, and also such things as religion, science, and mathematics. As far as health is concerned, it is worth looking at the heart line (see page 90), where it runs along the base of this mount, as this area relates to hearing and, to some extent, eyesight.

## The Mount of Apollo

If you want to improve your home or achieve creative success, this area will benefit from a massage. It also has important implications for love and relationships. As far as health is concerned, this mount relates to eyesight and, to a lesser extent, hearing.

## The Mount of Mercury

This relates to the brain—the ability to think and communicate—breathing, and some dental problems can show up here. The heart line starts under

Mercury, and if it is flaky or disturbed, this is a classic indication of heart problems, so massage this area frequently if this seems to be the case.

Look at the edge of the mount and see if there are any glassy warts there, possibly sitting within the little lines that form on the side of the hand. These indicate cancer, especially in the reproductive organs. Obviously, it will take more than a reflexology treatment to deal with this, but picking up this ailment at an early stage means the individual can get it treated sooner.

## The Mounts of Mars

There are two mounts of Mars, and strangely, the one by the thumb is called *Lower Mars*, despite being higher on the hand than the mount that's on the percussion side, which is called *Upper Mars*. Both speak of courage, with the first being the ability to get through the difficulties faced in childhood and youth, and the second being courage in general. If either mount is flat and thin, the person may be a victim of bullying.

These days, we tend to talk about someone having strong nerves or plenty of backbone if they are courageous, but long ago, courage was considered to come from the stomach. Unsurprisingly, Lower Mars concerns the digestion while Upper Mars is connected to the liver, gallbladder, and other organs of digestion, so massage both Mars mounts if your digestion isn't working properly or if you need a boost to your courage.

## The Plain of Mars

This is the center of the hand, so it acts like a crossroads. If anything is bothering you or if you feel off-color, give this area a massage.

## The Mount of Venus

As far as health is concerned, this area is devoted to strength and vitality and to sexuality. If you need to feel stronger, or you want to boost your sexual performance, focus on this area. Other matters related to Venus are comfort, luxury, possessions, money, and having the best of everything, so if you are short on these things, focus your reflexology here.

## The Mount of Luna

This area is hard to read, but a skilled palmist can pick up a dark patch that contains small flaky lines, which denotes diabetes. Another problem in this area is the breakup of skin-ridge patterns that talk of alcoholism. The area is also linked to memory, so if there are disturbances here, the mind may not be functioning perfectly. This mount concerns spiritual matters, but also travel and exploration. So, if these things are important to you, give this area a reflexology treatment.

## The Mount of Pluto

This is the lower end of the mount of Luna. It doesn't have any specific health problems attached to it, but if it is prominent, it shows extreme restlessness and a tendency to get bored easily.

## The Mount of Neptune

This refers to the reproductive organs, so a patch of redness or broken and disturbed lines in this area can indicate problems with the womb in women or the genitals in men. Lots of little flaky lines that suddenly appear on a woman's hand, coupled with a touch of redness, can indicate pregnancy. This mount is also the link between the material world of Venus and the spiritual world of Luna, so if it is prominent, it shows that the person can tap into spirituality to benefit others as well as benefiting him- or herself. Many people have hands that become red, especially around the percussion edge and the bottom of the hand. There are various reasons for this, including a problem with the thyroid gland or lung damage due to heavy smoking. Sometimes such redness signifies a quick temper, especially if the hand is thick through the percussion side. Whatever the cause, a reflexology treatment may help.

# The Lines on the Hand

The accompanying illustration shows the three major lines on the hand. The upper line is the *heart line*, the middle one is the *head line*, and the one going down the hand is the *life line*. These three are enough for our purposes. If any of

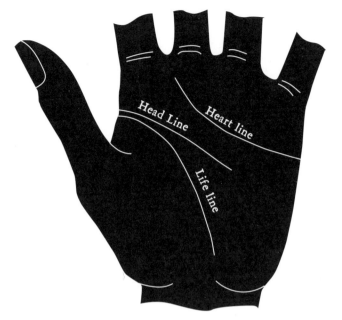

The major lines on the hand.

the problems that are linked to these lines are bothering you or those who you want to help, give the line a reflexology treatment.

## The Heart Line

This line starts at the percussion edge of the hand, and it can travel straight across the hand or curve upward in anything from a gentle to a deep curve. The deeper the curve, the more sensitive and romantic the individual, and this person may even become obsessed with loving someone who doesn't love them back. A straight line belongs to someone who is quite likely to marry the person they consider "suitable" for some reason or other, rather than because they have fallen in love. Emotionally speaking, islands along the line show upsets in the person's love life, and a break in the line talks of a broken heart.

As far as health is concerned, if the percussion edge becomes broken and flaky, the heart is becoming weak or damaged. If the line splits, forming an island under the mount of Mercury, there may be dental problems. Discoloration on the line can suggest bronchial problems. Disturbances on the heart line where it starts to bend upward under the mount of Saturn can be a sign of serious trouble in the lungs or breasts.

## The Head Line

This can run straight across the hand or bend downward. It can be a single line or it can be in all kinds of pieces. It is more likely to be smooth in a young person and disturbed in an older one, where life has left its mark.

A straight line that runs across the hand belongs to a practical person who may be good at making things or who may be good at business. This person may be into mathematics, science, farming, building, or anything else of a practical nature. A curved line shows an imaginative nature, which indicates a poetic mind, a love of music, or intuitiveness, and it may lead to creative or business success.

Pits and dots along the line mean headaches, while small, white islands can mean fluctuations in eyesight. If the islands are red, there will be a serious problem with the eyes. Larger islands under the mount of Saturn can indicate oncoming deafness. Large islands or breakups in the line suggest mental problems of some kind. A break with a square over it that seems to mend the break talks of an accident from which the person recovers. If the line becomes flaky toward the end, the person will suffer from some measure of dementia toward the end of life. If a line coming in from the side of the hand splits and looks like a pair of sugar tongs reaching for the end of the head line, that shows insomnia.

## The Life Line

This line shows strength, energy, and the ability to recover from illness, but it doesn't show the length of life, so if someone has a short lifeline, it points to a major change in the person's life rather than an early death.

If the line curves deeply into the hand, the subject is strong and vigorous but also strong-minded and unlikely to be pushed around. A straighter line shows weaker health and someone who has a busy mind rather than physical strength. This subject may not be very interested in money and possessions, but in things that give life meaning.

The life line represents the spinal column and the legs, with the neck at the top and the feet at the bottom. Any disturbance on this line—in particular, any pits or dots along the line—can talk of problems with the bones of the back, hips, legs, and feet. Other ailments will show up as breaks in the line,

# EAR REFLEXOLOGY

Ear reflexology is effective but it can only be done by a practitioner who has very small fingers that can reach the right spots on the recipient's ears. There are ninety-one points, and they cover various parts of the body. Ear reflexology can be used for pain relief, clearing infection, balancing hormones, and treating kidney problems, among many other things.

Below is a massage routine for the ear. It's described as a self-massage, but you can also perform it on another person.

- Sit upright on a chair.

- Keep an ear chart handy and find the reflex points you need to work on.

- Tuck your hair back, using a couple of hair clips to hold it in place.

- Gently tug the lobe of one ear downward while pressing it. Do the same with the other lobe.

- Run your finger round the edge of the ear and notice whether there are any areas that feel lumpy, crunchy, or crusty.

- Now work your thumb and forefinger over the outer part of whole ear, starting at the top and working downward. Press firmly but gently and note if there are lumpy or crunchy areas or areas that you find slightly sore. If so, note the body areas that these relate to and work on them for a while.

- Do the same with the ridges and valleys of the middle and inner parts of the ear. If it is hard to get your fingers to work on these areas, a cotton swab may do the trick.

- Repeat the process with the other ear.

- Wash your hands and pour yourself a drink of water.

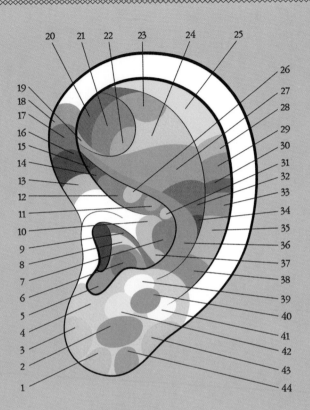

1. Cheek
2. Eye
3. Nose
4. Head
5. Lung
6. Heart
7. Liver
8. Trachea
9. Esophagus
10. Stomach
11. Pancreas
12. Intestines
13. Rectum
14. Bladder
15. Prostate

16. Ureter
17. Genitals
18. Anus
19. Sciatic nerve
20. Foot
21. Leg
22. Hip
23. Thumb
24. Hand/Palm
25. Fingers
26. Kidneys
27. Abdomen
28. Wrist
29. Lower arm
30. Elbow

31. Gall bladder
32. Chest
33. Upper arm
34. Clavicle
35. Shoulder
36. Spine
37. Spleen
38. Neck
39. Upper jaw
40. Tongue
41. Lower jaw
42. Mouth
43. Inner ear
44. Tonsils

long islands where the life line splits into two and then joins up again, lines that seem to act as a bar across the line, dark patches, and red patches. Many of these marks come and go as the health fluctuates.

## The Rascettes

The rascettes are lines that form on the wrists. If they are strongly marked, the person will be vigorous and long lived, but if they are weak and broken, the person will struggle with health problems. When the uppermost rascette loops upward into the mount of Neptune, this indicates problems with the bronchial tubes and the lungs, which may be due to asthma or heavy smoking.

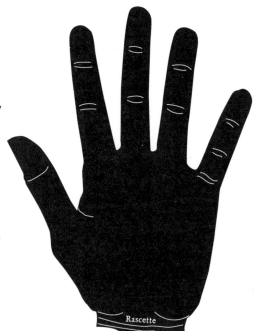

Rascette

## Red Patches

Red patches on any part of the hand mean trouble of a temporary nature. If they are on the palm side of the hand, this might be caused by a sudden health issue or perhaps an emotional matter that comes out of the blue, but it could also be something the person has brought on him- or herself.

Red patches on the backs of the fingers or hands are caused by the behavior of others, and you can see how they impact you by looking at the area of the hand that they appear on. Give any red patch a gentle reflexology treatment to help cope with the situation.

- If a red patch appears on the Jupiter finger or knuckle, someone is trying to undermine you and even to damage your reputation. Someone may be questioning the things you value and believe in.
- If on the Saturn finger or knuckle, there is worry about finances, security, business matters, or even something more abstract, such as your religion or beliefs.

- If on the Apollo finger or knuckle, there could be worry about your home and family, but it could equally be someone who is holding back something that you are trying to achieve. Redness here can also tell of a relationship problem or of love that isn't being returned.
- If on the Mercury finger or knuckle, there is difficulty in communication, either because someone in your life isn't hearing what you have to say or due to practical issues such as problems with telephones, computers, and so on. Your sex life may be stressful due to the way someone is treating you.
- If on the thumb, someone is trying to hold you back and to prevent you from doing the things you need to do. If the redness is on the lower joint of the thumb, this person will doubt your judgment or say you are being illogical.

The rest of the back of the hand is less important, but my advice is to pay attention to any red patches or dark patches that you see, because they may be linked to aggravation that is coming at you from other people in your life.

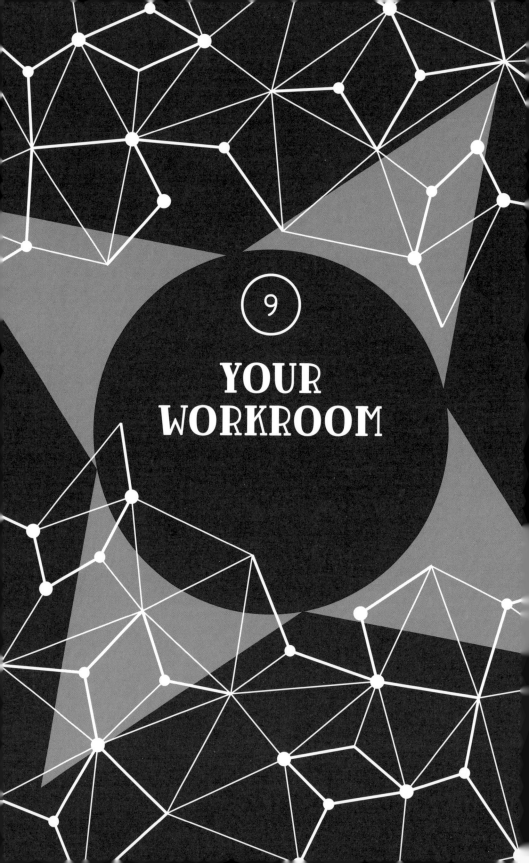

9

# YOUR
# WORKROOM

Once you have practiced on yourself, friends, and family, your confidence will have grown. Gradually you will remember which reflex zones relate to which part of the body. How the body is mapped out on the hands and feet will become second nature. Also, the more feet and hands you work on, the more you will be able to recognize common symptoms and issues.

After experiencing firsthand the multiple benefits of reflexology, you may want to become qualified as a practitioner so that you can provide this therapy to others. When you are working on yourself, all you really need is a willingness to learn and patience. You can make the space in which you do reflexology calm by using candles, burning oils or using a diffuser, and playing soothing music. As long as you have some comfortable cushions and a blanket or towel at hand, you are just about set to go. Even though you technically need very little to practice reflexology on yourself or your family, there are some basic equipment and guidelines that can help you create the perfect healing environment.


## Mindfulness

When we take the time to light candles, put on a diffuser, burn aromatherapy oils, and focus on our breathing, we instantly bring ourselves back to the present moment. This grounds us, helps us to let go of the past and not obsess about what may happen to the future. Being in the present moment is all we truly have, but convincing our ego and the negative voice we hear in our head takes a lot of practice.


## Setting the Scene

Setting the scene is important, whether it's for you to practice reflexology on your own hands or for another person who wants a reflexology treatment. You can dramatically improve your treatment room by creating a calm atmosphere, a haven from the outside world where individuals can step away from technology and leave their stresses and worries behind.

As soon as someone is with you, tell them this is *their* time. They may want to talk about how they feel, how tired, stressed, or overwhelmed they feel.

If they do, this is normal. Allow your recipients to unload their stresses and worries, and reassure them they are in a safe environment, and that the session is all about them. Encourage them to allow themselves to truly relax and be in the moment.

If you have the space, create a separate room for treatments and furnish it appropriately. Ensure there are no televisions or other screens in the room, but if you sometimes need to use the space as an office, cover any screens with a colorful throw. It's a good idea to shut out the outside world and light candles to create a low, soothing light in which to work. This way, the recipients' brains won't be overstimulated by light, and they can relax into their session. Making sure the room is warm will also help them relax. Ask recipients to remove watches and large jewelry in order to further reduce distractions.

Remember, if they drift off into a relaxed, semi-sleep state, they are likely to feel cold. Having a large pile of blankets close by is essential so that you can offer them or add layers if someone says they are getting cold. Make sure at the beginning of a session that all of your own technology is switched to do-not-disturb mode, and encourage the recipient to do the same.

## Questions You Need to Ask

There are several questions you should ask before beginning treatment:
- Are you pregnant?
- Are you a diabetic?
- Do you have a pacemaker?

### An Important Point
Only experienced and confident reflexologists should treat pregnant women, those with pacemakers, or diabetics. Pregnant women would enjoy a generalized foot massage, even without the reflexology element added.

# Creating the Ideal Atmosphere with Aromatherapy

Use an aromatherapy diffuser in the room to further enhance a healing, safe environment. It creates a cool mist that gently adds essential oils to the air and creates a soothing environment as well. Fan diffusers don't affect the chemical compounds of essential oils in the way that candles or heat diffusers can, so make sure you get a fan diffuser or a nebulizing or evaporative one. Many essential oils, especially bergamot and lavender, promote good sleep by stimulating the release of serotonin and dopamine. Others, such as lemon, tea tree, and eucalyptus, boost immune health and help eliminate coughs and colds. Lavender and bergamot can also help boost the mood, and for those feeling anxiety, frankincense, neroli, and chamomile can promote a calm body and mind. For people with low energy, grapefruit, cinnamon, lemon, and orange will boost energy and mood. For those working on weight loss, grapefruit, ylang ylang, patchouli, orange, and lavender can affect the limbic system (the emotional side of the brain) and help curb appetite. To improve cognitive function, diffuse rosemary, basil, lemongrass, tangerine, or spearmint.

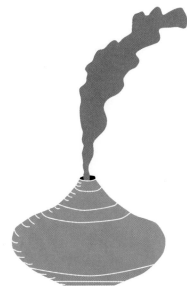

At the beginning of a session, ask your recipient what their main reason is for wanting to receive reflexology, and choose one of the above oils according to what they tell you. You can have a box on your couch and explain some of the benefits of the oils. Give the individual an opportunity to smell them to see if they're drawn to any one in particular, because their innate need for healing will guide them to the right oil.

## Conscious Color

Color is a communicator that can contribute greatly to creating a healing environment as it can greatly inspire moods. Essentially, it will inspire well-being from the outside in. If you have a treatment room, ask yourself: "How would I want someone to feel in this space?" Also, ask how *you* would like to feel in your daily workspace. Think of what you want the overall goal to be for your recipient: Is it to feel relaxed, safe, and calm? You can also draw from nature and outside environments that influence your mood. Do you find mountains or white sandy beaches relaxing? Or the moon and stars? Or sunrises or sunsets? Colors from all of these can be integrated into your working environment if you choose them.

The colors you use in your treatment room will set the tone of the work you do and will communicate well-being. Colors influence our emotions. In general, warm colors (red, orange, gold, and yellow) have a stimulating effect, whereas cool colors (green, turquoise, blue, and violet) are calming. Neutral tones such as cream, mushroom, and beige are a blend of warm and cool colors, and they have a balancing effect.

The colors you choose for your environment don't have to be overwhelming—you can use them sparingly to create a meaningful effect. The color turquoise can create an inspiring, opening, and giving atmosphere, whereas pale blue can create a calming, relaxing, and peaceful mood. Green is balancing, soothing, and caring; deep violet is meditative, centering, and wise; white is expanding, purifying, and open.

You can also customize your treatment space for different people you work on. Those areas that can easily be changed, such as towels, cushions, blankets, sheets, and your work clothes, could be adapted according to the needs of regular clients. The most important thing to remember is not to limit yourself. Colors have many hues, so the possibility of creating the perfect healing space is endless. Neutral-colored carpets and walls can be offset with beautiful images of forests and mountains, clouds, rivers, and waterfalls.

## Take Your Time

It's important at the beginning of a session to allow time for the person to transition into the treatment and the healing environment they have stepped into. Color, soft lighting, essential oils, warmth, calm music all help, but make sure they don't feel rushed. Always allow time to talk through the issues they want help with, what they hope to achieve from the treatment, and setting their intention—a short mantra of what they want to focus on in the session. If they have no specific intention they want to set, offer a simple one, such as "I am happy, healthy, and whole."

# Mindful Breathing

Once the person is settled, take a moment to help him slow down his breathing. Place your hands on the soles of his feet, and ask him to breathe in deeply for a count of four, and then out for a count of six. Doing this yourself at the same time can help guide the other person into deepening the breath. Spend a minute or so allowing the person to relax, and ask him to wriggle a bit and make sure he is really comfortable. Being comfortable helps recipients maximize the benefits of the session.

You can encourage the person to visualize inhaling the healing energy of the universe that surrounds him, and to imagine the way the oxygen that is traveling through his nose down into his lungs and body is being energized.

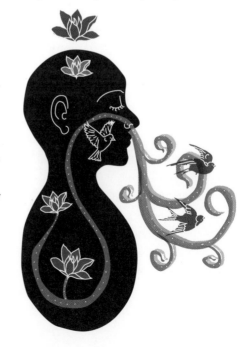

Ask him to truly focus on feeling the air in his nose and lungs so that he is connecting with his body. Ask him to feel the healing energy of the breath as it enters his body. On the exhaled breath, encourage the person to imagine breathing out any stress or worries. On each exhalation, ask him to let out the breath fully, right to the tip of exhalation. Encourage him to pause between each breath. Gradually he will let go of tension as he focuses more on the breath.

At the end of the treatment, return to your position with your hands on the soles of the feet, and again ask the person to focus on some deep breaths in and out. Again he can focus on breathing in calming, healing energy and, as he breathes out, letting go of any stress or worries. Some deep, gentle breaths at the end of a session will help the transition back to normal reality, as well as provide a positive ending.

Deep breathing has many positive benefits, including reducing stress, relaxing the body and mind, and promoting sleep. It is a natural painkiller because it promotes the release of endorphins, improves blood flow, and detoxifies the body. It will supercharge your recipient and allow him to return to his day energized.

Then give the person the opportunity to discuss what he felt during the treatment—if he wishes to. Ask him how the treatment felt and whether he had any particular sensations, thoughts, or emotions during the session, because these may reveal blocks in energy related to the physical blocks that you will have detected on the feet. Feedback will help guide you with the person's future treatments, as well as make you a better practitioner!

# Equipment

Now let's look at the basic equipment that you will need to start working with reflexology. You don't need to buy this equipment if you are working on family and friends, although you will probably find that once you start this therapy you will want to invest in a massage table. Relatively inexpensive, these fold up, are lightweight, and can easily be stored in a small space. Using a table will be more comfortable for you when you give a treatment to another person, but it is not an essential piece of equipment.

## A Reflexology Chair

You may need to buy a special bench-type chair that allows people to lie back while their feet are supported at the lower end. This will allow you to work on the feet in comfort. This piece of equipment is the most expensive part of the business, so you will need to search the Internet for reflexology organizations in your area to see what is available. You may be able to find some pre-owned equipment in your area or that is available to ship to you. An alternative might be a therapy couch, which is more likely to be available on the pre-owned market as there are many more of these available.

## Treatment Table

Reflexology equipment doesn't have to be expensive, but investing in a good treatment table will ensure comfort as well as protect from possible injury. Buying a table that is adjustable will allow you to set it to the right height for you to work at. Consider buying a secondhand table at first so that you can build your base before you pay out a lot of money for a brand-new table. You can buy a static table that doesn't fold up, but portable, adjustable tables will give you the ability to take reflexology into people's homes.

## Clothing

If you are going to become a professional reflexologist rather than just give reflexology to friends and colleagues, you should wear a special tunic of the kind that dentists and other therapists wear. This makes you look professional, and it saves your own clothes from getting cream or other stuff on them. You can find these on the Internet.

## Powder

When you perform reflexology, you will lightly dust the feet or hands with powder to help you grip the foot or hand and to ensure you have good control over your movements. Avoid talcum powder; instead, use corn flour or arrowroot powder. Also avoid using oil during a treatment as this will make it difficult to perform the correct technique. If you wish to massage the feet after the treatment has finished, you could use almond oil or coconut oil, which are light and less greasy than some other products. Some reflexologists choose to use aqueous cream, which is absorbed quickly.

## Cream

If someone has dry feet, you may want to end the session by massaging in some foot cream. Special reflexology creams that don't contain any aromatherapy material or perfume are available on the Internet, or you can buy a basic nonperfumed moisturizer in your local pharmacy or supermarket.

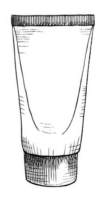

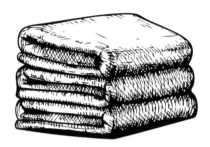

## Towels

Make sure you have plenty of towels at hand for recipients to lie on and to keep the feet warm. Also ensure that you have blankets within reach for people who feel the cold. Staying still for an hour can make some people feel chilled, which makes them tense.

## Additional Equipment

Make sure you have plenty of pillows at hand, and place one pillow under your recipient's knees to allow him to feel relaxed and comfortable.

Using an exercise ball, or a chair on wheels that can be easily moved around a treatment table, can make working with reflexology both easier and better for your back.

Relaxing music on low in the background can help people feel more peaceful and give them a nicer experience. Take care not to play a radio, though, or you could find yourself in trouble with copyright issues.

A jug of water and disposable cups should always be available so that the person you're working on can drink some water as soon as the treatment finishes.

Keep a box of tissues within reach.

# Comfort

Here is a basic checklist of things you can do to make sure the person you're working with feels comfortable throughout the session:

- Make sure the person doesn't feel rushed on arrival and knows where the water and tissues are.
- Ask the person to take off shoes and socks and settle on the treatment table.
- Offer pillows or cushions to help the person get comfortable—and provide a blanket if wanted.
- Suggest a pillow under the knees and behind the back to take any strain off the hips and lower back.
- Take a few moments to look at the person's feet. Check to see if there are any open sores or wounds, fungal infections, or rashes. If any

## Tip

If you are a beginner, you might want to keep a few reflexology maps on the wall of your treatment room, both for you to refer to and for the people you treat to look at. It may also be helpful to use a water-soluble pen to draw the diaphragm line and waist line on to the foot.

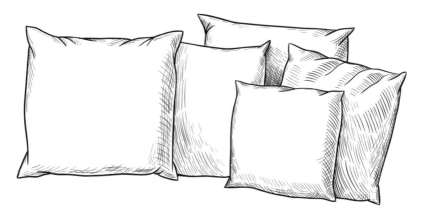

of these are present, suggest hand treatments until the issue has been resolved.

- Gently cover both feet with powder. Wrap one foot in a towel to keep it warm while you treat the other foot.
- If the person is feeling nervous or anxious, suggest some simple deep breathing to help him relax. Ask him to breathe in for a count of four, and then out for a count of eight. While he does this, you can begin to focus your attention on the treatment.

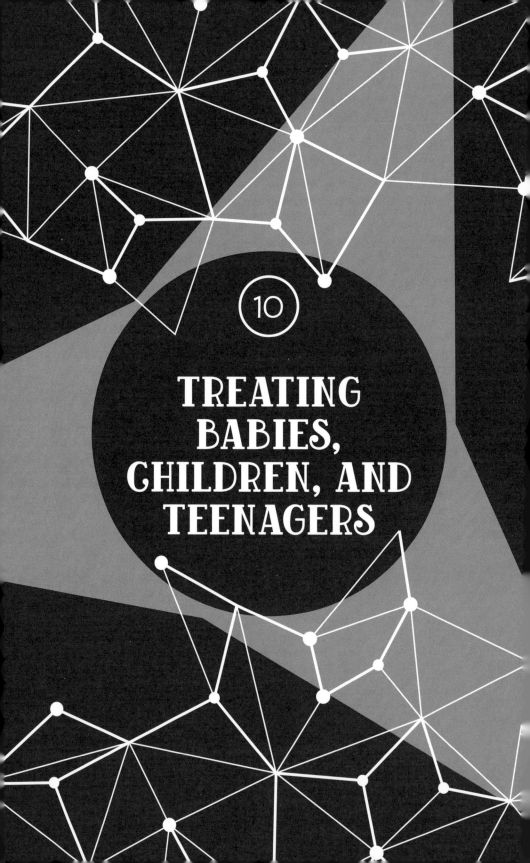

# 10

# TREATING BABIES, CHILDREN, AND TEENAGERS

Babies and children thrive from touch, and reflexology can be a wonderful experience for parents and children to share. Regular treatments can also boost the immune system and assist recovery from illness.

Babies are very sensitive to touch, and gentle treatments on tiny feet can not only help with common ailments such as colic and teething, but also help establish loving bonds. As babies and children receive loving touch, it will also help boost their self-esteem and awareness of the needs of others.

Many mothers will make a full body massage a daily part of their routine, especially after bath time and before bedtime. Just five minutes of gentle pressure over the whole of the foot will help baby settle.

## Tip

Seek medical advice if your baby has the following:

- A temperature over 102°F (39°C)

- Fits or seizures

- Labored breathing

- Diarrhea or vomiting

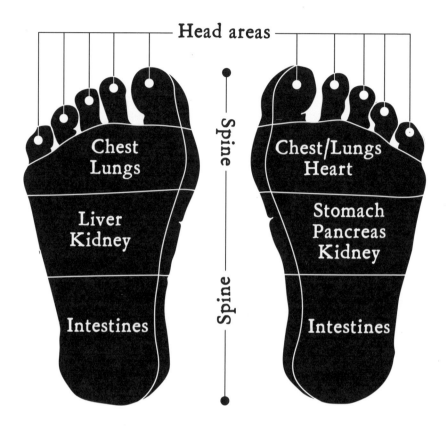

Foot map for an infant to three-year-old.

## The Foot Map for an Infant to Three-Year-Old

The arches of the feet develop slowly, so until the age of three the feet are oval in shape and this leads to a broad division of areas for treatment. Young feet are so small, it's easy to cover the whole foot several times during a treatment.

Start on the inside of the right foot and slowly work from the base of the heel upward to where the toes join the foot, with a tiny caterpillar movement of the thumb. Cover the whole of the foot toward the outside edge, and repeat on the left foot. This will cover all the energy zones.

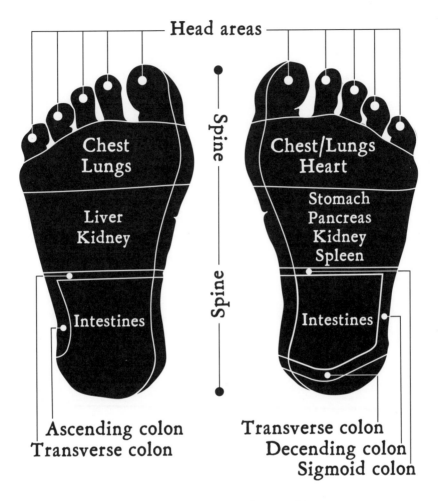

Foot map for a three- to five-year-old.

## The Foot Map for a Three- to Five-Year-Old

As the arches form by the age of about three, the shape begins to change. The subsequent narrowing of the foot allows the middle of the body to be worked on more easily, as it's now located on the narrowing point of each foot. The feet are still too small for specific treatment, but these maps show the general divisions.

\* \* \*

# Children's Ailments

The passage of childhood is often punctuated by illnesses and diseases. From teething and colic in babies, to eczema and asthma, fever, tonsillitis, the common cold, earache, night terrors, and bed-wetting, to chicken pox, measles, and other ailments—the early years are usually full of sickness. These can be troublesome for children to cope with, but will also greatly affect their sleep.

Regular reflexology doesn't claim to cure ailments, but it can help children get over them much more quickly and hopefully prevent regular occurrences. Treatment allows young children to relax deeply, boosting their immune system. The younger children are when they are introduced to reflexology, the more they will accept it. Giving time to children boosts their sense of self-esteem and nurtures their belief in their own worthiness. Making reflexology into a game by engaging children's imagination will allow them to lead the session. Ask them to tell you what they are thinking about as you massage their feet or to put into words what they are feeling. For example, if they have an earache, encourage them to imagine the pain in their ear shrinking to the size of a grain of sand, which they can then place on their hand and blow high up into the sky.

For a baby who is suffering from teething, a five-minute massage may help relieve their pain, improve circulation to the mouth and gum areas, as well as reduce inflammation. For a baby who has earache, gently massage the area of the foot beneath the instep in a circular motion. This will help calm the baby as well as help the healing process. When working on babies, make sure you always use light stroking rather than pressing.

For all the common childhood illnesses, reflexology will help children recover more quickly as well as boost their immune system so that hopefully they will suffer less from colds, earache, sore throats, and upset stomachs. Let's look at some specific ailments and techniques for soothing them.

## Sleeplessness

A baby or young child who is incredibly alert and active may make parents feel they have their hands full! Many babies and young children struggle to sleep through the night, with some not achieving this milestone until they start school around five years old. Gentle massage can help babies and young children relax and become calmer in the evenings. Even with infants, especially when they are agitated, you can gently hold their feet and massage them. It's

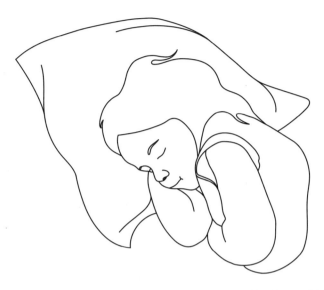

very important to have a clear evening routine with babies, which usually follows the format of bath, then massage, then bed. It is difficult working on tiny feet, but as a guide, focus on the reflex areas for the head, which means gently massaging the toes, especially the big one. Make up songs and games while you gently massage the feet to make this time fun.

Work on the balls of the feet to help calm baby's breathing, as well as under the ball of the foot to work the solar plexus, in order to encourage deep relaxation. With babies and children, unless they fall asleep immediately, it's sometimes hard to tell if the massage is successful, because they can't communicate what they are feeling. But establishing a sacred routine not only allows parents and babies precious time together in a busy household, it also encourages babies to prepare for nighttime. It also helps parents to try to stay relaxed and calm at a difficult time of day when they themselves are tired. Parents may find, even as their children get older, they will ask to have their feet or hands rubbed when they're feeling poorly or when struggling with an issue. Reflexology is more than just a chance to help children relax and heal; it also gives them the opportunity to feel safe and talk about their feelings, and this is priceless.

## Soothing Earache

Earache is a common childhood ailment. If you're looking for a more holistic approach to helping soothe the symptoms of earache in children, reflexology can help.

For children, having a constant earache can make it harder for them to understand what people are saying to them; they will often struggle to hear their schoolteachers. Having an earache can also make it difficult to concentrate. It can cause children to feel angry as it is painful and frustrating, like having a bad headache all the time. Going to sleep becomes difficult as well, as they often cannot stop thinking about the pain.

Reflexology can help ease the pain of an earache. Children will find the massage relaxing, and it can often make them feel sleepy, especially if the pressure isn't too hard, but more importantly it can help to calm them down so that any angry feelings they may have from the pain don't overflow. You can work on the ear reflexes and the solar plexus, diaphragm, and chest in order to encourage relaxation. There are also reflexes for the inner ear, neck, throat, upper and lower jaw, and cervical spine, all of which can provide some relief from symptoms and help children's bodies find a balance that will boost healing.

# Psychological Boost

Today's technological society means that children grow up accustomed to screens, are exposed to global events, and feel judged. Reflexology need not be used only to help children overcome any physical problems they experience—emotional well-being is as important as having a healthy body, and children need to be educated on the importance of talking about their feelings without the fear of punishment.

If a child is finding something difficult, just being able to talk may help them process their problems. Whether it's a problem at school or home, taking the time to massage their feet provides them with the opportunity to discuss what is troubling them. Time together with the family is vitally important, but it has been eroded with the advent of social media and multimedia. Reflexology can bring families together in a nonthreatening experience, giving them time to talk to each other. Touch is so crucial to human beings, especially young people. Skin-to-skin contact is essential to babies and children as it shows them they are safe, and builds trust between child and parent. It is this contact that encourages development and recognition of self, cognitive skills, and emotional competency.

With babies and children, it's important to keep sessions short, so aim for ten minutes. And make sure they have fun!

# Dealing with Bullying

Bullying can make a child very anxious, which can be distressing to see in someone so young. Many children who are bullied completely close down and won't talk about what they are experiencing or their feelings. It's very easy for children who suffer from bullying to believe they are worthless. Reflexology allows children to be able to relax and also provides a good chance to talk. Start with a long warm-up massage in each session to help the child relax, and allow them to talk about any problems during the massage. Never force children to talk, only allow them the opportunity. If at first they are reluctant, ask them to think about anything they may want to talk about during their next massage.

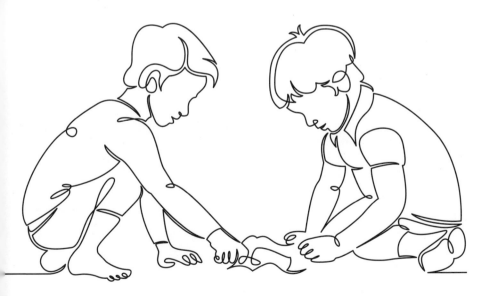

If you are able to specify a problem that they would like to discuss during the massage, you will probably find that by the time you have finished with each foot, the child will have come up with some solution that works for them. It may take a few sessions to really open up about how they feel about being bullied, but setting this time aside will soon become a time for you both to talk about any issues that came up. Reflexology will continue to help the child relax and let go of worries, but it will become so much more than this, because by talking about how they can tackle new problems, it allows them to come up with their own solutions, which boosts their self-esteem.

# Working with Teenagers

We can all remember how stressful being a teenager is. Teenagers can feel a lot of pressure, due to social media, expectations from their family, peer pressure, and pressure from teachers. They also have to deal with hormonal stress, which can affect their sleep patterns. Giving teenagers a coping strategy, such as reflexology, can provide them with a way out from the constant feelings of anxiety and pressure. Teenagers may be reluctant to try a complementary session such as reflexology, so they may feel nervous and anxious when they first try it. It's important to put them at ease and establish a calm environment, away from the outside world and the ever-present social media that is part of the world they have grown up in.

Teenagers may present with constant feelings of stress, fearing failure in exams, feeling stressed about being judged for who they are or what they do. It's important to listen to their worries and support them without judgment. At the beginning of the session, talk through exactly what is going to happen to put them at ease. Once you start massaging their feet, they will feel even more at ease.

Encourage teenagers to work out their own simple coping strategies; often, talking to an adult who is not part of a

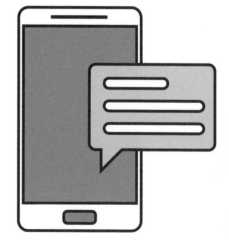

family will help them gain perspective and work out their problems. For teenagers with stress headaches or shoulder, neck, and back ache, work on the spine reflexes. The biggest benefit of a reflexology session to teenagers is that it will help them feel deeply relaxed. It will improve their sleep and be a great stress buster, especially during exam time. It can help balance their endocrine system, helping them cope with the normal hormonal imbalances they are experiencing. For girls who are beginning their periods, it can help alleviate pain.

Introducing this therapy to teenagers will also encourage them to take an active role in taking care of their own health in the future.

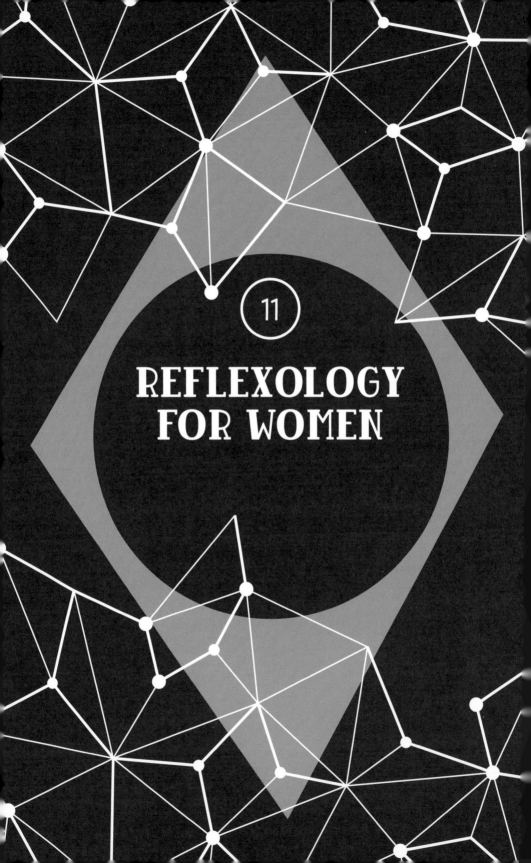

11

# REFLEXOLOGY FOR WOMEN

Reflexology can help with a range of common health issues that women suffer from. Not only can it offer a safe haven away from the daily stresses of life, it can also help balance the body's systems.

## Reflexology and Fertility

Stimulating the reflexes in the feet for the endocrine glands and reproductive organs can help restore balance in these systems as well as promote better health. Stress can affect the reproductive system, but a series of reflexology treatments, over a period of time, can help the mind and body to relax.

Reflexology may also help relieve symptoms associated with endometriosis, polycystic ovary syndrome, and irregular periods. It can regulate hormones, increase blood flow, boost the immune system, and reduce premenstrual and menstrual problems. Promoting a deep sense of relaxation counters the effect of too much cortisol (the stress hormone) in the body, and can have an immediate impact, improving sleep as well as helping alleviate menstrual or fertility problems.

## Reflexology and Breast Cancer

Research has shown that reflexology can help cancer sufferers manage their symptoms and perform daily tasks more easily. It has become one of the most popular complementary therapies used by women who have cancer, due to its helping on three levels. First, it helps women to relax and cope with the stress and anxiety caused by living with cancer. Second, it relieves pain. Finally, it can lift their mood and enhance their feelings of well-being.

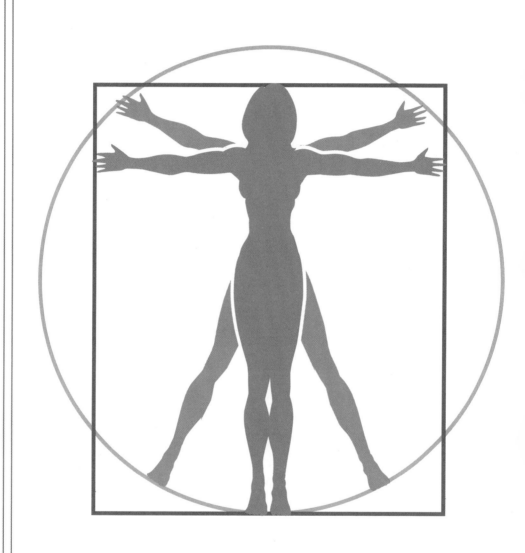

## Reflexology and Stress

As reflexology calms the nervous system, it can help us cope with our busy lifestyles when we find ourselves constantly worried, or in a "fight or flight" state. Such a state heightens the levels of cortisol in our body. Cortisol is designed to regulate blood pressure and the immune system in a crisis. Many women today suffer from consistently high levels of cortisol due to the enormous pressure they feel they are living under. This directly affects sleep, but it can also impact the immune system and cause insulin resistance and weight gain.

## Reflexology and Menopause

Women usually start experiencing menopause symptoms between forty-five and fifty-five years of age, as their estrogen levels decline. For some women, though, this can occur much earlier, in their thirties, whereas others may continue to have periods into their late fifties or early sixties.

Menopause affects all women, but individually the experiences may differ vastly. Typical symptoms, which are caused by a natural dip in estrogen levels, include hot flashes, night sweats, vaginal dryness, difficulty sleeping, low mood, anxiety, reduced sex drive (libido), and problems with memory and concentration. For some women, these symptoms last several years, but for others they may continue for up to fifteen years.

As women approach their late thirties, their ovaries start making less estrogen and progesterone—the hormones that regulate menstruation—and fertility declines. In their forties, during perimenopause (the time leading up to the last period), women's menstrual periods may become longer or shorter, heavier or lighter, and more or less frequent, until eventually, on average, by age fifty-one, the ovaries stop producing eggs and the woman has no more periods.

Estrogen plays a role in body temperature regulation, which helps to explain why hot flashes and night sweats occur. Declining estrogen can explain changes in skin and hair. Changing hormone levels may also cause mood swings and other emotional changes. The impact estrogen and progesterone have on the body is widespread, and research continues to be done to better understand the roles these hormones play.

These hormonal changes occur naturally, but they can be exacerbated by poor lifestyle choices, smoking, excessive alcohol, poor diet, lack of exercise, and so on.

The hot flash is well known as the classic menopausal symptom. (British women call these hot *flushes* rather than flashes.) Hot flashes and sweats are called *vasomotor symptoms* and vary immensely in both their severity and duration; for many women, they occur occasionally and do not cause much distress. However, for about 20 percent of women, they can be severe and can cause significant interference with work, sleep, and quality of life.

As a woman's estrogen declines, alongside other contributory factors, the thermostat in the brain malfunctions so that it thinks the body is overheating when it isn't. This leads the brain to switch on cooling mechanisms such as sweating and blood flow through skin blood vessels (flush) to dissipate heat. The sensation varies from one woman to the next, as does the severity, duration, and frequency of the hot flash. Hot flashes usually last between three and five minutes. If they occur at night, they can disturb the woman's sleep, which can then have secondary effects on energy and mood.

Normally, there is a daily pattern of rises and falls in body temperature, with the temperature being lowest at about three a.m. and highest in the early evening. These small changes are not normally noticed, but a menopausal woman may flush with every temperature rise, whether these are normal changes or not—for example, moving between areas of different temperature or having a hot drink.

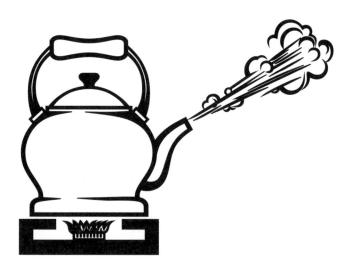

Hot flashes can also be associated with headaches and palpitations. Approximately 85 percent of women are affected in some way by these early-onset symptoms, which can be to manage or adapt to.

Reflexology can help make the symptoms of menopause more bearable. Many of these symptoms are caused by stress and worry that occur due to the hormonal changes in a woman's body. Reflexology can help the body release and regulate the hormones and improve the glandular functions of the body. It can also help control the body's emotional and physical balance. It can improve circulation in the reproductive areas as well as balance energy. By working with the hypothalamus and pituitary, reflexology can help to restore balance to the endocrine system.

Other simple steps, like wearing loose layers of cotton clothing rather than man-made fibers, and having a fan in the bedroom can help during hot flashes. Excess caffeine can worsen palpitations, so menopausal women who drink coffee, tea, and caffeinated soft drinks should do so in moderation.

## Menopause and Insomnia

Many menopausal women experience sleeping problems, including insomnia, oversleeping, or difficulty staying asleep. As menopause can be a time of major hormonal change for women, it's natural to expect some disruption to the normal sleep routine. Declining levels of estrogen and progesterone can have a drastic impact on sleep. Estrogen is important for managing the level of magnesium in the body. This is a chemical that allows muscles to relax, so low levels make it difficult to fall asleep. Lowered levels of progesterone make it more difficult to slip into deep sleep. Even if the sufferer doesn't wake during the night, her sleep isn't as restful as it should be. Sleep problems can be very disruptive, leading to daytime drowsiness, and are often accompanied by anxiety or depression. They may also cause the woman to have trouble concentrating during the day.

The deep relaxation that reflexology promotes will help reduce insomnia as well as help balance mood. It can give a woman a safe space to relax, and by calming the central nervous system, it can alleviate anxiety and stress. It can also help the ovaries regulate their secretion of estrogen and maintain the health of the uterus.

## Menopause and Change in Mood

For many, changes in mood can be just as debilitating as the physical symptoms. Research has shown that 61 percent of women suffer anxiety during perimenopause. Many, however, are unaware that they may be in the perimenopause phase of life and that changing hormone levels may be responsible for their change in mood.

Perimenopausal women may find themselves experiencing low mood, anxiety, inability to concentrate, forgetfulness, low self-esteem, and feelings of fatigue—or several of these symptoms at once, leaving them feeling exhausted by being on this hormonal "roller coaster."

Reflexology is a wonderful way to lift the mood. It induces a deep state of relaxation, as well as encourages the release of endorphins, which are the feel-good hormones. It can help perimenopausal and menopausal women feel calm and confident. So, if you are giving reflexology while this is ongoing, encourage the woman to take some deep breaths, for the count of four inward and then a count of four outward, and to center herself. During inhalation, ask her to visualize energy moving into her body, and during exhalation visualize breathing out a black cloud that floats away, far up into the universe, with all her problems going up, up, and away with the cloud.

Another way to lift someone's mood is exercise, which leads to the production of endorphins, and being outside enhances this effect. Avoiding alcohol, which can trigger low moods, is another option. Many pharmaceutical and medical experts in the UK also back the use of the herb St. John's wort to treat mild depression—but this cannot be taken in conjunction with some other medicines.

## Tip

You must not take St. John's wort when you are using certain medications, so read the instructions that come with your medications and also with the St. John's wort before using it.

## Menopause and Loss of Libido

Loss of libido is a complex phenomenon with psychological, relational, physical, and hormonal dimensions, as unique as the women who experience them. It is chiefly characterized by a lack of interest in or desire for sexual activity. Many women who lose their libido find that they lose touch with their sexuality. Sexual feelings and desires come less frequently, and the energy required for sex drastically dwindles or disappears from a woman's life. Reflexology can't stop the natural process of the menopause, but it can help ease the effects on the hormonal systems and promote a sense of well-being while a woman's body changes. It can also help a woman to relax physically, to let go of worries and reduce tension throughout the body.

During menopause, even if a woman may not want to have sex, asking her partner to massage her feet can feel nurturing without making her feel pressured. If she decides she does want to have sex, a foot massage may help her feel more responsive and open. It's the ideal way to communicate without talking. It allows partners to provide relaxation and to make a physical connection. It can be a way that both people can show their love for each other. It's also an opportunity for partners to loosen up and relax together during stressful times. When we are relaxed, we often feel more confident about expressing ourselves, so reflexology can also allow couples to open up and communicate, building feelings of trust and closeness.

If you or your partner is going through menopause, book a reflexology date night, where you can use a session to get to know each other again. Taking time to massage each other's feet can help improve communication, and simple touch may help to boost libido. Make sure the mood of the space is right, with low lighting and relaxing music. Switch off phones and other electronic devices so that you can give each other your full attention.

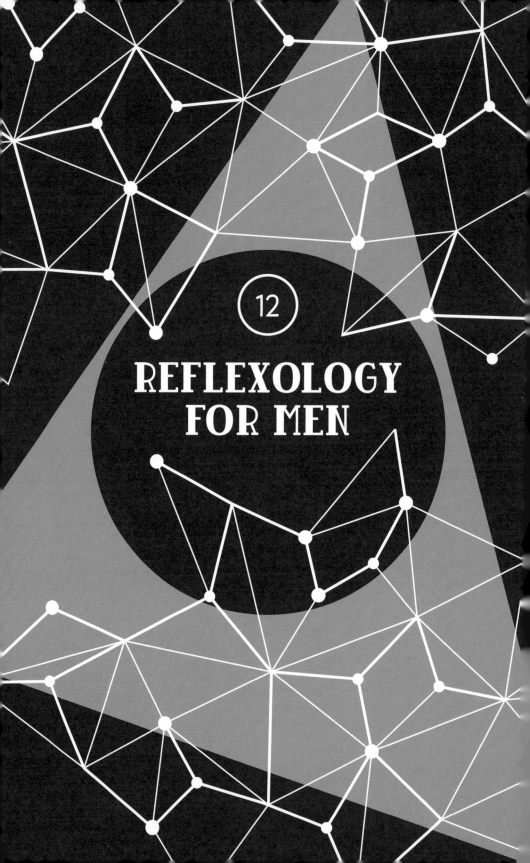

## 12

# REFLEXOLOGY FOR MEN

Reflexology can benefit anyone, regardless of sex. Many complementary therapies are traditionally sought out by women, however, reflexology has a myriad of benefits for men.

Many men don't actively seek out complementary therapies, just as they often don't make the trip to their doctor as quickly or regularly as they should—this is known as "avoidance behavior." Statistically, women are better at seeking health and medical support than men. It's often a case that men come to complementary therapies through receiving a gift or being encouraged by their partner to give these therapies a try.

As with trying all new things, people who are coming to reflexology for the first time might be skeptical of it. Another barrier for many—women and men—is the inherent awkwardness of having someone else touching their feet. When faced with this initial skepticism and awkwardness, you need to gently reassure the person you are helping. It's surprising how quickly this feeling will evaporate once the treatment begins, and you will soon be happily chatting with each other.

## Helping with Stress

For a man who works full-time, has a family, juggles all the commitments of life as well as finds time to keep up his hobbies such as sports, it's likely that his feet get little respite. Some professions are more demanding than others, such as construction, and for these men a reflexology session allows them a small window to literally put their feet up and relax. A treatment can help relieve achy feet, as well as help to reduce overall stress. Promoting a sense of relaxation will also have a secondary effect on sleep; just like after a yoga class when a person experiences the best night's sleep ever, having a reflexology treatment promotes much deeper sleep. Poor sleep patterns can result in a reduced immune function, as well as increase irritability and stress. Reflexology can be viewed as a first positive step toward a new, healthier, more balanced lifestyle.

The nervous system is triggered during reflexology, helping to restore the body to a state of calm, and through this deep state of calm, the body is able to allow itself to rest, restore, and recover. A deep sense of relaxation doesn't just benefit the mind. The secondary effects are that other systems, such as the

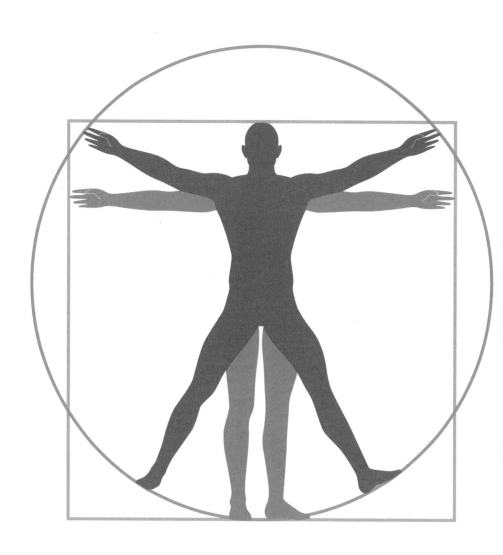

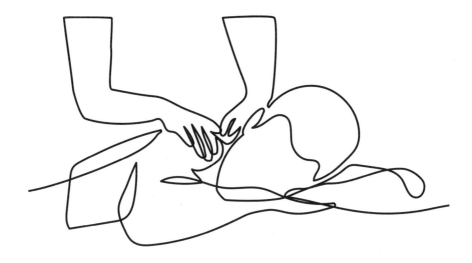

digestive system, become more relaxed. Stress hormones are reduced and blood pressure is lowered, which can also help a person make better decisions.

## Helping with Anxiety

Men suffer from anxiety, stress, and depression as much as women, even if traditionally women have been slightly ahead of men in discussing mental health issues. Men live in the same fast-paced world as women and struggle with the same responsibilities, worries, and fears. The feelings of being overwhelmed that mothers experience as they juggle family, home, and work are also experienced by men, juggling the same situations. And yet traditionally, men are much less likely to reach out to friends or family if they are suffering from mental health issues. For those men who prefer not to discuss their feelings, a reflexology treatment gives them vital time and space to stop, ground themselves, and focus on the present. Taking one hour a week to pause from their daily schedule, stop, and focus on the breath and the present moment will allow mind and body to rejuvenate.

## Reflexology and Sex Drive

Loss of libido is a common problem that affects many men at some stage in their life. Increased stress, depression, fatigue, anxiety, relationship issues, or underlying medical problems can all affect sex drive. If lack of desire for sex is affecting a man's relationship, or is causing anxiety, reflexology can help.

If stress is the main underlying reason for loss of libido, turning to something unhealthy, such as drinking, won't help. Reflexology can help manage stress, make the person feel back in control of his life, and help him to be more positive. The opportunity to stop and rest can help clear a person's thoughts so that they can deal with problems more calmly. It may help ease some of the emotional intensity a man has been experiencing.

Relaxing the mind and releasing tension in all parts of your body also allows people to be more responsive and sensitive to sexual pleasure. Working the reflex points of the brain, hypothalamus, pituitary, and the reproductive system can stimulate hormone production and help get men and women in the mood!

## Reflexology and Sexual Dysfunction

Premature ejaculation and impotency are common sexual problems in men, with stress being a major factor. This stress can be tackled positively with reflexology, which helps promote deep relaxation. Couples reflexology is preferable, where each person spends thirty minutes on their partner's feet. Not only are both people respecting each other's need to relax, they are nurturing each other through encouraging their partner's body to heal. This therapy can help encourage positive emotions toward each other, as well as intimacy—often the first thing to be dropped when tired from looking after family as well as working. It also allows partners to feel more self-confident in expressing needs. Practicing reflexology offers a safe environment to talk about true feelings.

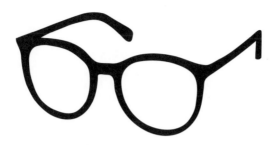

## Other Common Problems

Another problem that is common in men is acidity in the stomach that can lead to stomach ulcers. These can benefit from reflexology, both directly by helping the stomach to work properly and indirectly by the relaxation the treatment gives.

Just about everybody—and every man who has ever lived—suffers from backache from time to time. The spinal reflex lies along the inner side of the sole, and it is easy for a man to massage this area himself when he is relaxing in front of the television or after a bath or a shower. If he is in a relationship, he could ask his partner to do this for him as an act of loving kindness. A visit to a reflexologist could be a real help easing the pain of muscular strain in the back.

A man who spends his day working on a computer may suffer from tired eyes or eyestrain. Obviously, he must consult an optician about this, and he may need to use drops for dry eyes, but a reflexology treatment may be helpful for this minor ailment.

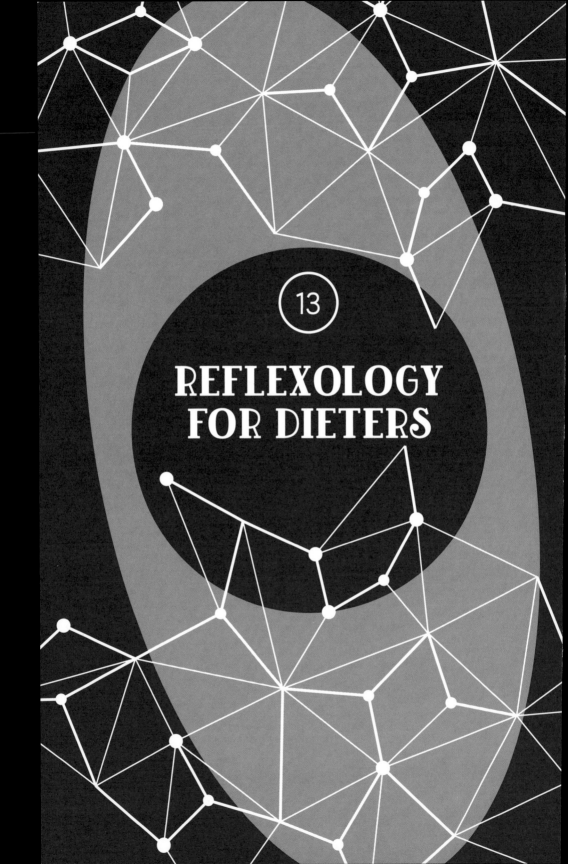

13

# REFLEXOLOGY
# FOR DIETERS

It seems as though just about everyone in the Western world is on a diet these days, struggling to keep their weight in check when surrounded by so much temptation. For those who are overweight, reflexology won't bring about a miracle but it may help, especially when conducted alongside other steps, such as following an online weight-loss regime, joining a diet group, or simply substituting healthy snacks for fattening ones. Clinical research doesn't support reflexology as a weight-loss method, but it is known to reduce stress, so perhaps that's why it helps people lose weight.

## Tips

- A good night's sleep aids relaxation, relieves stress, and therefore helps dieters stay on track. Reflexology can definitely help with this.

- You can also use hand reflexology on your own hands to keep the stimulation going between visits to your reflexologist.

## The Stomach and Pancreas

The stomach point is on the inside arch of the foot, just under the ball of the foot, and the pancreas reflex is in the middle of the arch of the foot. Stimulating these points improves digestion and encourages the recipient to eat better-quality food. Cradle the person's left foot with your right hand and press the reflex point with your left thumb. When you reach the outside limit of the reflex area, switch hands and work the reflex points back in the opposite direction. Repeat on the other foot.

## Stimulating the Spleen

Stimulation of the spleen reduces hunger, so try this: Support the person's left foot with your right hand and use your left thumb to work the spleen reflex.

## The Gallbladder

The gallbladder area is a small point in the liver reflex area on the right foot. This is just below the ball of the foot, near the outside of the foot. Like the stomach and pancreas, this area can be encouraged to prompt the person you're working on to eat well and digest food properly. The gallbladder stores bile, which is the digestive liquid continually secreted by the liver, and it emulsifies fats in partly digested food, which aids weight loss.

## The Endocrine Glands

The thyroid gland reflex is at the base of the big toe, and the pituitary gland reflex is in the center of the lower part of the big toe. The adrenal gland reflexes are between the waist line and the diaphragm line. Together, these are the endocrine glands.

The endocrine glands regulate the response to stress, so applying pressure to the reflex points for the thyroid gland, pituitary gland, and adrenals will help balance emotional and physiological stress. The less stress the person is under, the better he or she will cope with dieting and may feel more inclined to exercise as well.

* * *

## Hand Reflexology for Weight Loss

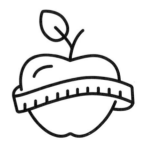

Hand reflexology can be useful for those who want to lose weight, and it works well when it's not possible

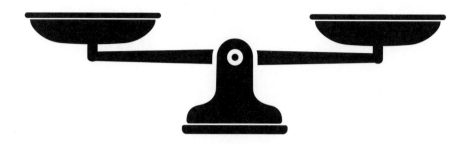

to get to a reflexologist for a full foot treatment. Press a little more deeply than you would for the feet, and keep the pressure up for a little longer. The hands are smaller than the feet, so take care to cover the right reflex areas and move slowly along them in tiny steps.

Find the reflex area for the spleen, which is located below the little finger on the left hand, and work that. Now work the digestive organs, which are beneath the lung and breast area on both hands; the gallbladder area, which is on the mount or pad under the little finger on the right hand; and finally the endocrine glands, which have reflexes on the middle and lower areas of the thumbs on both hands.

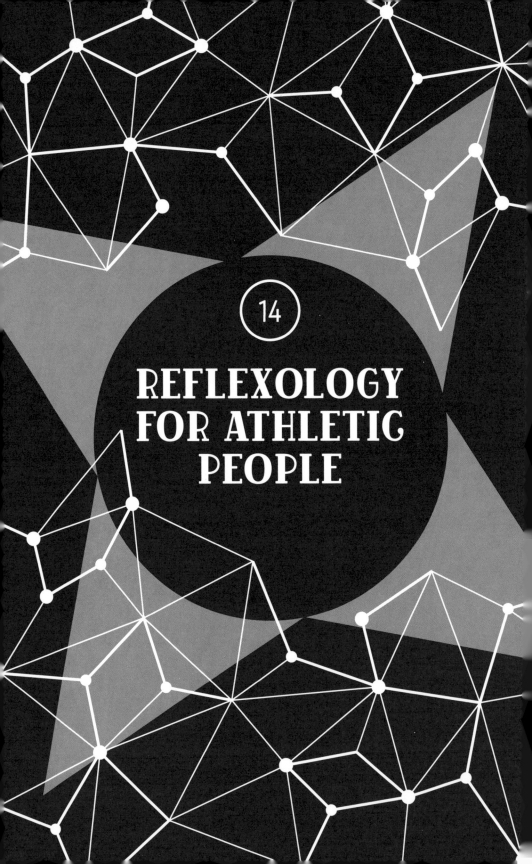

14

# REFLEXOLOGY FOR ATHLETIC PEOPLE

Whatever sport a person participates in, reflexology can have a positive impact on performance, speed up recovery from injury, and improve emotional and physical health by helping to reduce pain as well as encourage overall relaxation. Whether a person is a social jogger, a semi-pro cyclist, a professional basketball player, or participates in sport to keep fit and healthy, incorporating reflexology into the training regime will bring huge benefits. We all know that to be successful in a sport, people need to balance their physical, mental, and emotional selves. Reflexology promotes balance in the body and will become a vital tool in their training tool box.

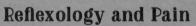

## Reflexology and Pain

Reflexology can help to reduce pain, such as knee pain or foot pain caused by tendonitis or plantar fasciitis, without resulting in invasive surgery or the need for drugs. For the athlete, this often results in less recovery time and thus less time away from their sport. It is just as beneficial for sports that stress the shoulders, arms, and hands such as tennis, golf, and basketball. For those with a painful injury on the foot, reflexology on the hand can be used. Whatever the specific injury is, look at a map of the feet or hands and work on the reflex area that relates to that body area. For muscle pain, work on the reflex related to the muscle area affected. Also work on the adrenal reflex to stimulate anti-inflammatory hormones, and on the lungs and chest reflexes, to improve circulation and heal the affected area.

## Reflexology and Recovery

Research has shown that reflexology can remove lactic acid from the legs four times faster than massage, thereby helping relieve leg pain following high-impact sports. For athletes who are suffering from DOMS (delayed onset muscle soreness) due to a high-impact session, having reflexology will promote recovery in their muscles. This means they will be able to return to training sooner. By increasing blood flow, reflexology removes toxins from the blood, promoting faster recovery. It also stimulates the transportation of essential oxygen, nutrients, minerals, enzymes, and hormones to the muscles. Think of it this way: the system gets a physiological boost, which energizes tired muscles. Increased circulation can assist in preventing cramps, spasms, aches, and pains associated with extended exercise. Working on the lymphatic, neck, chest, and groin reflexes will stimulate the removal of waste from the muscles.

## Reflexology and Relaxation

Reflexology helps to de-stress and relax the body, mind, and spirit. Acute, short-term stress may be beneficial to an athlete as it helps to increase adrenalin; too much stress, however, may result in tight muscles or reduced function in the cardiovascular system. Following a reflexology treatment, muscles feel looser and improved blood flow helps to ensure the cardiovascular system is brought into balance. Athletes who are competing in a major event should plan their reflexology treatment two to three days in advance to allow the body to eliminate toxins and regain a state of balance.

Work on the adrenal reflex to stabilize energy, the pancreas reflex to balance blood sugar levels, the diaphragm to increase relaxation, and the lungs and chest reflexes to deepen and regulate breathing.

## Reflexology and Sleep

Reflexology encourages the body to fall into a deep state of relaxation, which often results in an improvement in sleep patterns following treatments. Sleep helps to ensure the body returns to its natural balance and relieves muscle tension or pain due to injuries. Too much exercise can impact sleep, so reflexology can prevent this from becoming a problem. People who participate in sports, more than anyone, rely on being physically and mentally alert. Most athletes will tell you they struggle to sleep well the night before an event, game, or competition. Getting into a relaxed state will help them sleep more soundly and perform when it really counts. The reflex areas to work are the solar plexus, diaphragm, pineal gland, pituitary gland, and brain.

# Reflexology and Performance Success

Having the best physique, the sharpest mind, and determination will not alone win an athlete an Olympic medal. Athletes who stay focused on the present and the immediate challenge they face, while ignoring negative self-talk and avoid replaying past mistakes, are the ones who don't break when the pressure to perform mounts. Going into a sporting event feeling rested and relaxed gives an athlete an edge over their competitors. Managing stress, and other marginal gains, can help make an athlete into a champion. Therefore, it's crucial to improve sleep and ease tension leading up to a sporting event. Stress and tension tighten the cardiovascular system and restrict blood flow, causing it to become sluggish. This results in the tissues becoming oxygen-deprived; the energy in the body becomes depleted, making all body systems suffer. The practice of reflexology, by stimulating the nerve endings on the feet, keeps the body's circulation flowing smoothly, rejuvenating tired tissues and promoting a sense of balance, calm, and wellness. For highly competitive sports, it is best to have reflexology two or three days before an event, to allow the body to achieve a state of balance.

Whatever sport an athlete participates in, reflexology sessions can be easily incorporated into their weekly routine or training plan and will become as essential as their regular sports massage. Reflexologists can show athletes what reflexes to work on, and how to do massage on their own feet, so that they can top off their treatments if needed, helping them achieve optimal physical and emotional well-being.

❋ ❋ ❋

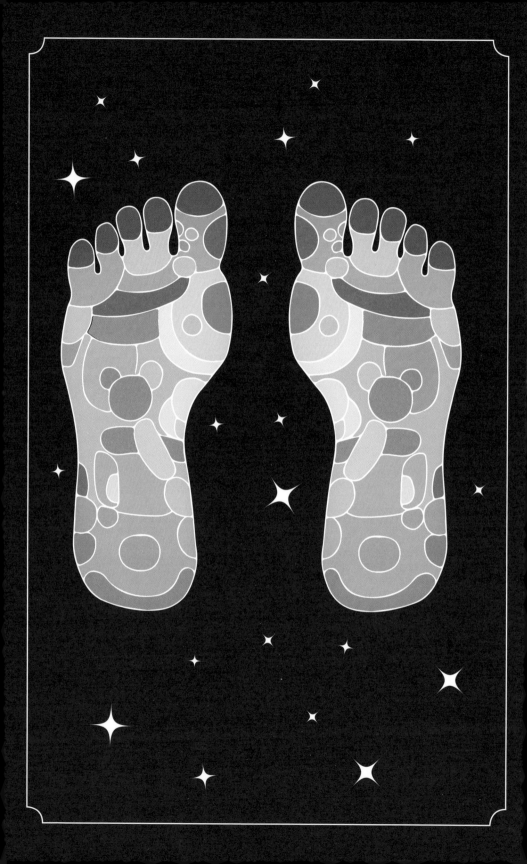

# CONCLUSION

Reflexology is for everyone. It can greatly improve health and well-being as well as ease symptoms of pain and discomfort. It can be practiced easily, without great expense, and it provides the vital healing touch that can work alongside traditional medicine to boost your health and the health of other people. Reflexology can easily be used in the home or the workplace, on the feet or the hands. Babies and octogenarians can benefit from this complementary therapy; the power of touch is a global method of healing. Learning the methods of giving reflexology is easy, and it can provide wonderful effects to the people you treat.

Reflexology can also enhance your own healing as it can easily be applied to yourself. Giving, and receiving, treatment can also be very rewarding. When trying this therapy, give yourself time to respond, as it can often take up to six treatments for benefits to be felt. If you are inspired to take up reflexology professionally, try a treatment from a qualified reflexologist to get an insight into how a session evolves and what it feels like to receive this therapy. Then contact the reflexology association in your country to find an accredited teacher in your area.

The healing benefits of reflexology are matched by the deep state of relaxation it promotes. Together, these can bring a wonderful sense of inner peace for all.

# ABOUT THE AUTHOR

Tina Chantrey, BA (Hons) in History, MA in Media Studies, Cirf (England Athletics Coach in Running fitness), is also qualified as a massage therapist, reflexologist, and Reiki practitioner. She is the fitness editor of *Women's Running UK* magazine and, before this, was editor of *Women's Running* and deputy editor of *Running Fitness* magazine. She regularly writes for health, fitness, and outdoor women's publications.

Tina is the award-winning blogger *shewhodaresruns*. She has completed many marathons, half marathons, duathlons, and adventure races all over the world. In 2017 Tina qualified to represent Team GB in the European Duathlon Championships, and she reached the top 50 in the UK in her age group at numerous running distances.

Recently her work has appeared in *The Guardian, The Daily Express, Outdoor Fitness, Running, BBC Sport, Top Sante, Women's Health,* and *The Divorce Magazine,* and she has contributed to the *This Girl Can* campaign, as well as numerous podcasts and radio interviews. She regularly coaches women in her local community to run better and believe in themselves.

Tina's last book, *The Divorce Survival Guide: How Running Turned My Life Around,* was published in 2017 by Zambezi Publishing Ltd.

# IMAGE CREDITS

# INDEX